EDITED BY
Dr. STANISLAS F. SNIESZKO
and
Dr. HERBERT R. AXELROD

# DISEASES OF FISHES

This book is the second in a series of textbooks dealing with diseases and parasites of fishes.

## BOOK 2A: BACTERIAL DISEASES OF FISHES

GRAHAM L. BULLOCK, DAVID A. CONROY,*
AND S. F. SNIESZKO

## BOOK 2B: IDENTIFICATION OF FISH PATHOGENIC BACTERIA

GRAHAM L. BULLOCK

Bureau of Sport Fisheries and Wildlife
Eastern Fish Disease Laboratory
Kearneysville, West Virginia 25430

*Research Fellow, Fish Pathology
The Zoological Society of London
Regents Park
London N.W.1
England

Distributed in the U.S. by T.F.H. Publications, Inc., 211 West Sylvania Avenue, P.O. Box 427, Neptune, N.J. 07753; in England by T.F.H. (Gt. Britain) Ltd., 13 Nutley Lane, Reigate, Surrey; in Canada to the book store and library trade by Beaverbooks, 953 Dillingham Road, Pickering, Ontario L1W 1Z7; in Canada to the pet trade by Rolf C. Hagen Ltd., 3225 Sartelon Street, Montreal 382, Quebec; in Southeast Asia by Y.W. Ong, 9 Lorong 36 Geylang, Singapore 14; in Australia and the South Pacific by Pet Imports Pty. Ltd., P.O. Box 149, Brookvale 2100, N.S.W., Australia; in South Africa by Valiant Publishers (Pty.) Ltd., P.O. Box 78236, Sandton City, 2146, South Africa; Published by T.F.H. Publications, Inc., Ltd., The British Crown Colony of Hong Kong. Printed in Hong Kong.

# Contents

## FOREWORD

Fish culture is at present an important and rapidly expanding enterprise all around the world. In the developing countries, fishes are being raised as food, while in the more sophisticated nations, fish culture directs its energies primarily to restocking streams, lakes and rivers with "sport" fishes. But raising fishes for food, as is being done on the new catfish farms to be found in the mid-south of the United States, has taken on a new impetus even in developed nations. In Florida, Hong Kong, Singapore and Bangkok, tropical fish farming is an extremely important part of the local economy.

With the increasing demand for fishes for human food, *mariculture*, or fish farming, both in freshwater and saltwater, is rapidly expanding. In the United States, for example, production at private fish farms raising catfish, trout and aquarium fishes is now more economically important than fish culture for sport.

There is a great demand in North America for bait fishes because of the great abundance of waters in which sports fishing is possible. Bait fish culture is a multi-million dollar industry in the United States; raising goldfish, koi and warmwater aquarium fishes is at least a $12,000,000 business on the farming level (1969).

The most recent branch of mariculture has seen advances in raising fishes in brackish, estuarine and bay water in which marine, anadromous and catadromous fishes have successfully been grown and maintained. In addition, there is the annual production of hundreds of millions of salmon in the Soviet Union, Japan, northern Europe and the Pacific Northwest of the United States. Totally, fish production is a multi-billion dollar industry which involves many of the nations of the world.

It is not surprising, therefore, that there has been an increasing demand for knowledge about the nature and control of fish diseases. Intensive, efficient culture of any plant or animal requires crowding the organism more densely than it exists in nature. Under abnormally crowded condition, fishes often fall prey to communicable diseases which might reach catastrophic proportions. It is doubtful that any fish farm in the world has not yet suffered a major disaster due to an uncontrollable situation dealing directly with the health of the fishes.

The importance of accumulating and documenting the knowledge relating to fish diseases need not be stressed when you consider the importance of training people to recognize, treat and control diseases of fishes. Adequately training people without textbooks is inefficient and expensive, and the fishing industries of the world would be poorly served were skilled fish pathologists not enthusiastic about sharing their knowledge and experiences.

The purpose of this textbook is to provide modern, reliable information on fish diseases to teachers, researchers and students and to the increasing number of persons entering this new and rapidly growing field of veterinary medicine.

In discussions between Dr. Stanislaus Snieszko and Dr. Herbert R. Axelrod, a series of books dealing with various aspects of fish diseases seemed to be the practical answer to getting a cooperative effort accomplished between some twenty-odd specialists. Dr. Snieszko contacted experts in each and every division of the discipline we know as fish pathology, selecting only outstanding scientists who were willing and able to produce a "chapter" on their particular area of competency. Naturally some scientists had smaller areas than others; some were very busy at the time and some had more free time to devote to the task, so the remaining chapters might take a few more years to complete. But each chapter will be published in book form, as a separate entity, and sometime in the far-distant future the whole undertaking will be brought together into one great textbook of fish diseases.

At least this is the objective of Axelrod and Snieszko, two gentlemen who would hardly settle for anything but top quality work.

Workers who have a particular field of specialty and are considered very competent in their particular fields should contact either Dr. Snieszko or Axelrod through the publisher if they are willing to participate in this worthwhile and needed project.

# *Introduction*

The intent of this chapter is to review the information concerning various aspects of the bacterial diseases of fishes. The discussion will be directed more toward cultured rather than wild fishes, and to the freshwater rather than the marine environment. The reader is referred to the recent works by Sindermann (1966, 1970) for a detailed review of bacterial diseases of marine fishes. The principal fishes to be covered are the freshwater and anadromous salmonids, catadromous eels, the cultured pondfishes, and aquarium fishes when they are affected by the particular disease under discussion.

Fish disease investigators are well aware of the difficulty in deciding which species of bacteria are true fish pathogens. Some pathogens like *Aeromonas salmonicida* and *Hemophilus piscium* are not known to occur in the aquatic environment when fish are not present and they are considered true pathogens. Many of the common saprophytic water bacteria such as *Aeromonas liquefaciens*, *Pseudomonas* spp., myxobacteria and vibrio may produce disease when fishes are under stress from specific but poorly understood environmental conditions, which affect the susceptibility of the fish, growth rate and pathogenicity of the bacteria, or both. Disease production in fishes is similar to the process in other animals in that it is more complicated than mere contact between host and pathogen, and is dependent upon at least three factors: host susceptibility, pathogen virulence, and environmental conditions (Snieszko, 1958, 1964). Since each of these factors may be varied together with, or independently of, the other two, a large number of situations is possible. For example, if a population of fish is resistant to furunculosis, either from immunity or genetic factors, contact with the causative bacterium, *A. salmonicida,* probably will not result in disease. However, this same population of resistant trout may become infected and diseased if they are stressed by poor environmental conditions, such as incorrect water temperature, crowding, low oxygen, and the like. The ubiquitous water bacteria which constantly surround fish usually produce disease only when the fish are stressed by poor environmental conditions. A correlation has also been noted between the incidence of kidney disease (*Corynebacterium* sp.) and water chemistry (Warren, 1963a). For a better understanding of not only what types of bacteria can infect fishes but also the method of disease production, more work will have to be done on the modes of pathogenesis of the various reported pathogens. Some work has already been carried out and will be described in the appropriate sections.

In addition to the bacteria which infect, cause disease, and may kill fishes, there are those organisms which reside in fishes and use them as vectors to produce disease in other animals. Important human pathogens such as *Clostridium botulinum* (Bott, Deffner, McCoy, and Foster, 1964) have been isolated from fishes in the Great Lakes while *Leptospira* spp. have been shown to invade goldfish (Maestrone and Benjaminson, 1962). Various serotypes of *Escherichia coli* were isolated from fish in a Pennsylvania stream (Glantz and Krantz, 1965).

The practice of eating raw fish in Japan has led to many infections in human beings caused by *Vibrio parahaemolyticus* which on occasion may also cause disease in fish.

In order to show taxonomic relationships among the fish pathogenic bacteria to be discussed, they have been grouped according to the latest edition of *Bergey's Manual of Determinative Bacteriology* (Breed, Murray and Smith, 1957) (Table 1). Needless to say the listing is not complete but contains most of the reported diseases. Not all of the named species appear in the latest edition, but they are, at least for the present, the unofficial accepted nomenclature used by most fishery workers.

The generic and specific names of fishes have been taken, if included, from the American Fisheries Society *List of Common and Scientific Names of Fishes from the United States and Canada* (Bailey, 1960).

TABLE 1. Classification of fish pathogenic bacteria.

1. Order Pseudomonadales
   - Family Pseudomonadaceae
     - *Aeromonas salmonicida*—furunculosis
     - *Aeromonas liquefaciens*—hemorrhagic septicemia and other septicemic diseases (*A. punctata* and *A. hydrophila* are synonyms)
     - *Pseudomonas fluorescens* and closely related species—hemorrhagic septicemia and other septicemic diseases
   - Family Spirillaceae
     - **Vibrio anguillarum*—septicemic diseases in marine and some fresh-water fishes
     - * *Vibrio parahemolyticus*—enteritis in human beings and septicemias in marine fishes

* Species not established, or species not officially accepted in present edition.

2. Order Eubacteriales
    Family Brucellaceae
        ⋆*Hemophilus piscium*—ulcer disease
        ⋆*Pasteurella piscicida*—white perch pathogen
    Family Achromobacteraceae
        ⋆*Flavobacterium* sp.—infection in black mollies
    Family Corynebacteriaceae
        ⋆*Corynebacterium* sp.—kidney disease
    Family Lactobacillaceae
        ⋆*Streptococcus* sp.—infection in catfish
    Family Enterobacteriaceae
        Unclassified agent of redmouth of trout in western United States
        ⋆*Paracolobactrum anguillimortiferum* from eels
3. Order Myxobacterales
    Family Myxococcaceae
        *Chondrococcus columnaris*—columnaris disease
    Family Cytophagaceae
        ⋆*Cytophaga psychrophila*—coldwater or peduncle disease
    Myxobacteria (unclassified)—associated with gill disease
4. Order Actinomycetales
    Family Mycobacteriaceae
        *Mycobacterium fortuitum*, *Mycobacterium platypoecilus*, *Mycobacterium marinum* } Fish mycobacteriosis
    Family Actinomycetaceae
        *Nocardia asteroides*—nocardial infections in marine and freshwater fishes
    Family Streptomycetaceae
        ⋆*Streptomyces salmonicida*—streptomycete infection in salmon

# *Furunculosis*

## Introduction

Furunculosis is probably the best known and very widely distributed bacterial disease of cultured fishes, especially salmonids. Two excellent complete reviews cover many aspects of the disease and the causative agent (McGraw, 1952; Herman, 1968). Additional information can be found in the very detailed reports of the British Furunculosis Committee (Mackie, Arkwright, Pryce-Tannatt, Mottram, Johnston, and Menzies, 1930, 1933, 1935).

TABLE 2. Status of furunculosis in various countries (Herman, 1968)

| *Country* | *Status* | *Source* |
|---|---|---|
| Australia | Unreported | Snieszko, 1967, pers. comm. |
| Austria | Reported | Fijan, 1967, pers. comm. |
| Bulgaria | Reported | Kabaivanski *et al.*, 1954 |
| Canada | Isolated from wild fish | Rabb and McDermott, 1961 |
| Czechoslovakia | Reported | Dyk, 1953 |
| Denmark | Widespread | Christensen *et al.*, 1963 |
| England | Common in salmon kelts | Smith, 1962 |
| Finland | Probably present | Ojala, 1963 |
| France | Enzootic | Solacroup, 1963 |
| Germany | Enzootic | Liebmann, 1963; Deufel, 1967 |
| Hungary | Unreported | Fijan, 1967, pers. comm. |
| Ireland | Present in salmon | Hewetson, 1962 |
| Italy | Enzootic | Ghittino, 1963 |
| New Zealand | Unreported | Snieszko, 1967, pers. comm. |
| Poland | Sporadic | Kocylowski, 1963 |
| Scotland | Common in salmon kelts | Smith, 1962 |
| Sweden | Spread since 1951 | Ljungberg, 1963 |
| Switzerland | Unreported since 1958 | Matthey, 1963 |
| Rumania | Unreported | Fijan, 1967, pers. comm. |
| U.S.A. | Prevalent | Post, 1965 |
| U.S.S.R. | Unreported | Bauer and Uspenskaya, 1959 |
| Ukraine | Reported | Fijan, 1967, pers. comm. |
| Wales | Common in salmon | Smith, 1962 |
| Yugoslavia | Reported | Fijan, 1967, pers. comm. |

## Historical

The disease was originally described in 1894 and the bacterium causing it was isolated from diseased hatchery trout in Germany (Emmerich and Weibel, 1894). Furunculosis has since been reported from most parts of the world where salmonids are cultured (Table 2). The first description of furunculosis in the United States was in brook trout (*Salvelinus fontinalis*) in a hatchery in Michigan (Marsh, 1902). The disease was also reported from wild fish populations as in whitefish (*Prosopium williamsoni*) and dolly varden trout (*Salvelinus malma*) in the Elk River, Fernie, British Columbia (Duff, 1932) and brown trout (*Salmo trutta*) in the Madison River, in Montana (Fish, 1937).

There are two theories regarding the origin of furunculosis in America. The first is that the disease was brought in with infected brown trout from Germany, while an opposing view is that furunculosis was present in America and originally infected rainbow trout (*Salmo gairdneri*) in the western U.S. from which area it spread to the eastern U.S. and other parts of the world (Fish, 1937). This species has always been the most resistant of the trouts to furunculosis which indicates a possible previous exposure to the disease.

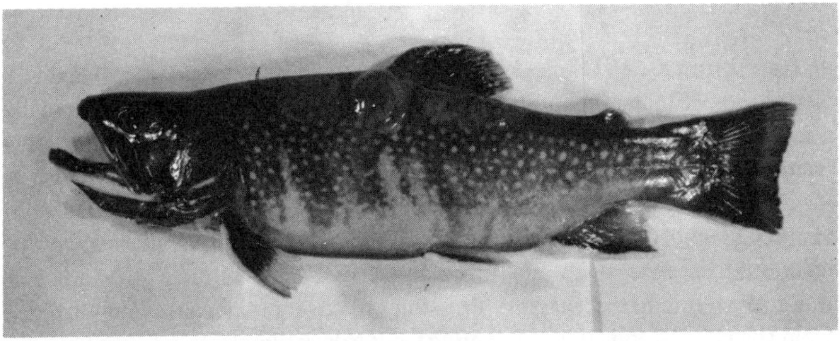

Figure 1. Adult brook trout (*Salvelinus fontinalis*) showing typical furuncle which may occur in chronic furunculosis.

## Symptoms and Pathology

Furunculosis is a generalized septicemia in which lesions termed furuncles (Fig. 1) may be produced if the disease does not progress too rapidly. When they occur, furuncles are formed as a result of bacteria collecting in the capillaries, where they multiply rapidly causing destruction of the walls of the blood vessels. The bacteria then move out into the muscle tissue where they continue to grow, producing a swollen area containing bacteria, blood,

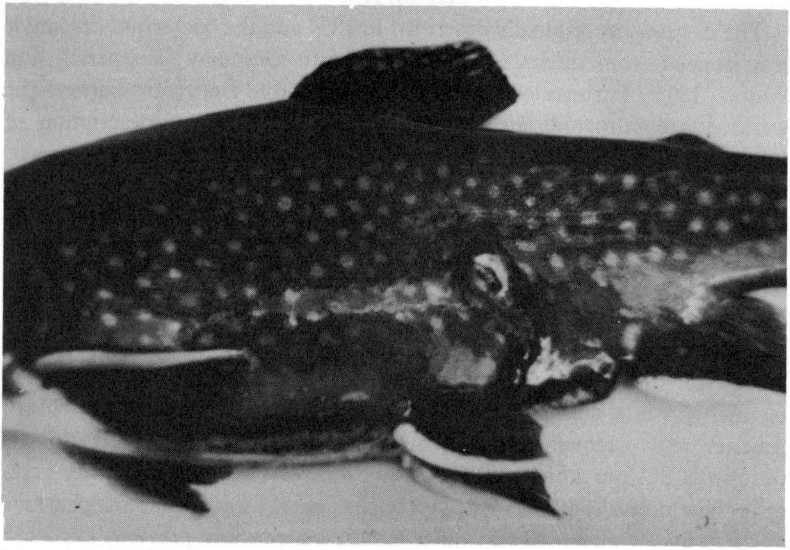

Figure 2. Adult brook trout (*Salvelinus fontinalis*) showing necrotic lesion from chronic furunculosis. (This figure, reproduced in color, appears after Index.)

and necrotic tissue (Davis, 1953). The furuncle may break open leaving a large lesion (Fig 2). It should be noted that the term furunculosis is actually a misnomer since no true furuncles are formed and the lesions contain only bacteria and necrotic tissue. However the name should be kept because of its long usage (McCraw, 1952). An enlarged cherry-red spleen is a convenient diagnostic character in fingerling trout. The gill capillaries may be congested because of clumps of bacteria. In Pacific salmon, gills are pale due to systemic hemorrhaging. Pressing gill covers may cause flow of blood from the gills (Wood, 1968). In young trout a dark blotch often forms between the pelvic and dorsal fins (Davis, 1953). However both the external and internal signs of the disease will vary depending on such factors as severity of the epizootic, susceptibility of the fish, and virulence of the pathogen.

Several disease forms of furunculosis have been described and those given by Herman (1968) encompass some of the more common symptoms.

Acute: sudden increase in mortality with few or no external gross symptoms.

Subacute: gradual increase in mortality with furuncles and hemorrhages at the base of fins.

Chronic: low steady mortality with intestinal inflammation and variable lesions.

Latent: no mortality, but the pathogen present systemically.

Many investigators have described internal pathology which has been summarized by McCraw (1952). Pathological changes include tissue necrosis in the kidney with accumulation of bacteria in the glomeruli; dark and enlarged spleen, petechiae in muscles, integument, peritoneum, and swim-bladder; and a flaccid inflamed intestine with a bloody discharge from the vent. A critical histological study of trout artificially infected with furunculosis revealed changes in several tissues when compared to uninfected trout (Klontz, Yasutake and Ross, 1966). One of the most interesting findings of the study was that contrary to many reports of an apparent lack of leucocytic response to the pathogen, there was such a response, but it was repressed within fifty-six hours after injection of the bacteria. Between forty-eight and fifty-six hours the hematopoietic activity of the kidney had virtually ceased. The liver was quite actively producing lymphocytes and macrophages, and the spleen appeared inactive and degenerate. The changes in the kidney and spleen became progressively more pronounced, and moribund trout had hematopoietic tissue in the anterior and mid-kidney completely destroyed. The spleen appeared fibrotic due to loss of follicular structure and the lymphocytopoietic activity in the liver had begun to decline. No significant abnormalities were noted in sections of stomach, pancreas, large intestine, or gill lamellae. These pathologic changes in artificially infected trout showed close correlation with pathologic changes in tissues made from trout with natural outbreaks of furunculosis.

## Etiology

The causative agent of furunculosis is a gram-negative, asporogenous, non-motile rod, which ferments selected carbohydrates and produces a brown water-soluble pigment when grown on the proper medium. The bacterium was known also as *Bacterium truttae* (Marsh, 1902) and until recently was classified as *Bacterium salmonicida.* After determining the characteristics of ten strains isolated from fishes from various parts of the United States, the organism was reclassified as *Aeromonas salmonicida* (Griffin, Snieszko and Friddle, 1953a). Other investigators also concluded that the furunculosis organism belonged in the *Aeromonas* genus because of its biochemical and serological similarities to the motile aeromonads (Ewing, Hugh and Johnson, 1961; Eddy, 1960, 1962; Karlsson, 1964; Liu, 1961; Bullock, 1966). However, Smith (1963) proposed that on the basis of computer analysis of strains of the furunculosis bacterium enough differences exist between *A. salmonicida* and the motile aeromonads that a new genus, *Necromonas,* be established for *A. salmonicida.* Pigmented strains would be *N. salmonicida* and non-pigmented strains would be *N. achromogenes.* Diagnostic characteristics of *A. salmonicida* are described in *Identification of Fish Pathogenic Bacteria.*

## Diagnosis

Positive diagnosis of furunculosis on the basis of gross symptoms is usually not accurate because many of the gram-negative fish pathogens such as *A. liquefaciens* and *P. fluorescens*, produced similar gross pathology. Presumptive identification of *A. salmonicida* is made on the basis of gram stain, motility and pigment production (Griffin *et al.*, 1953b, c), while positive identification is made on the basis of biochemical and serological tests described in *Identification of Fish Pathogenic Bacteria.*

## Transmission and Pathogenesis

Most workers agree that natural infection occurs from fish to fish through the gut or a mechanical break in the skin, however several assumptions have been offered to explain pathogenesis of *A. salmonicida.* The Furunculosis Committee (Mackie, *et al.*, 1935) felt that the pathogenic action of the bacterium was due to its abundant growth in tissues which interfered with blood supply and resulted in necrosis of the tissue. Other workers (Field, Gee, Elvehjem, and Juday, 1944) showed a rapid decline in blood sugar in trout with acute furunculosis which might induce a fatal hypoglycemic shock. The most recent studies on pathogenesis (Klontz *et al.*, 1966) have shown that *A. salmonicida* has an intracellular leucocytolytic substance which, when extracted from the cell with saline and injected into trout, produces almost the same changes as the entire bacterium. These workers postulated that in an actual infection the bacteria initially become localized and produce the leucocytolytic substance which destroys the inflammatory response and a fatal bacteriemia is produced.

## Host and Geographic Range

Of the eastern salmonids the brook trout (*S. fontinalis*) is the most susceptible; the brown trout is intermediate, and the rainbow trout is the least susceptible. However, great differences in susceptibility exist among strains of brook trout (Wolf, 1954; Snieszko, Dunbar and Bullock, 1959). The Atlantic salmon (*S. salar*) is also susceptible. Furunculosis has been reported in most of the western salmonids, however it was not reported in chinook salmon (*Oncorhynchus tshawytscha*) until 1959 (Wood, 1959). In Europe, it was found that among salmonids susceptibility to furunculosis increased with age, however, in the United States fingerling and yearling trout seem to be the most susceptible (McCraw, 1952).

In addition to salmonids furunculosis has been reported in many other species of fishes including: lamprey (*Ichthyomyzon castaneous*), perch (*Perca flavescens*), carp (*Cyprinus carpio*), catfish (*Ictalurus* spp.), pike (*Esox lucius*), sculpins (*Cottus* spp.), goldfish (*Carassius auratus*), whitefish (*Coregonus pollan*), tench (*Tinca tinca*), and various aquarium fishes (McCraw, 1952; Herman, 1968; Axelrod, 1962; Shechmeister, Watson, Cole, and Jackson, 1962). In general, it may be stated that probably most of the freshwater fishes can contract the disease under specific conditions. With the exception of Australia and New Zealand, furunculosis usually occurs wherever salmonids are cultured (Table 2).

## Control

Control of furunculosis can usually be accomplished by a combination of preventive and chemotherapeutic procedures. Preventive measures include: sanitation; manipulation of environmental conditions, breeding resistant fish; immunization; and prophylactic chemotherapy. Chemotherapy with sulfonamides, antibiotics and nitrofurans has been effective in controlling outbreaks of furunculosis.

## Prevention

*Sanitation.* Sanitation is the most important long-range control of furunculosis. If a population of trout at a hatchery is free of furunculosis and the water supply does not contain fish which carry the disease, strict sanitary measures should be used to stop the introduction of the disease with incoming eggs or fish.

Eggs coming into a hatchery should be disinfected and several methods have been discussed (McCraw, 1952). In any method used certain procedures should be followed to obtain the desired results. Even though eggs can be disinfected from fertilization to the eyed stage, they are most tender during the early development stages so that they may be handled best soon after fertilization. Before disinfection, eggs should be washed to remove organic material which may interfere with proper action of the disinfectant. They should be handled gently and agitated during treatment to expose all surfaces to the disinfectant. Also proper aeration should be provided during treatment. After disinfection, care should also be taken to discard and destroy clouded or dead eggs since these may harbor pathogenic bacteria.

The two most commonly used chemicals are acriflavine (Trypaflavine) and thimerosal (Merthiolate). As summarized by McCraw (1952), several investigators have suggested the use of acriflavine for disinfecting trout eggs. However it was found that the bacteriocidal activity of acriflavine is reduced in acid solutions and only solutions at pH 7.0 or above killed *A. Salmonicida* in 20 minutes (Smith, 1942). Therefore the disinfectant should be dissolved in water which has a pH at or above 7.0 (7.0–7.5) to obtain maximum benefit. After washing, eggs are transferred to a suitable container and a solution of 1:2000 acriflavine is poured in at the rate of 104 milliliters for each 1000 eggs and allowed to remain for twenty to thirty minutes. Eggs should be gently agitated each five to ten minutes to expose all surfaces. The solution should be periodically replaced with fresh disinfectant.

It was subsequently found that sulfomerthiolate was much more toxic to *A. salmonicida* than acriflavine without being toxic to eggs (Gee and Sarles,

1942). For treatment, eggs are transferred to a suitable container such as an enameled pan and a 1:5000 solution of sulfomerthiolate is poured in and the eggs are gently agitated every two minutes to expose all surfaces. Treatment should last for ten minutes and 50,000 eggs can be treated with 10 liters of solution (Snieszko and Friddle, 1948). Although the original experiments were carried out with sulfomerthiolate, this chemical is no longer available and is replaced with thimeorsal (Merthiolate). Experiments carried out at the Eastern Fish Disease Laboratory (Snieszko, 1953) have shown that thimeorsal is equally effective and is now recommended. The disinfectant should not be exposed to direct sunlight. In addition to disinfecting the eggs, care should be taken to disinfect the egg cases and to burn or disinfect egg packing material since these may contain the furunculosis bacterium. Anything which comes in contact with eggs or egg cases should be thoroughly disinfected to avoid spread of the furunculosis bacterium. Any recontamination of disinfected eggs makes the procedure of disinfection useless.

If fish are brought into a hatchery from an area where furunculosis is known to occur, these fish should be quarantined until they can be shown to be free of furunculosis or until they can be placed in raceways or ponds which are away from other fishes. If at all possible, every attempt should be made to obtain fish from areas free of furunculosis. However a hatchery water supply may contain fishes which are carriers of furunculosis or other diseases and even with the strictest sanitary procedures the bacterium may not be kept out of the hatchery. In such cases sanitation practices can be reinforced by using strains of trout resistant to furunculosis.

*Environmental conditions.* Probably of as equal importance as sanitation is the maintenance of conditions favorable to the fishes, such as adequate dissolved oxygen, correct water temperature, removal of waste and avoidance of crowding. As noted earlier, fishes resistant to furunculosis, which are carriers may become diseased if stressed. A correlation has also been noted between low oxygen levels and outbreaks of furunculosis (Kingsbury, 1961). The importance of stress conditions as contributory factors in epizootics will be more fully discussed in another section of this book.

*Resistance.* Selective breeding of trouts to obtain resistance to furunculosis has been carried on for many years (Embody and Hayford, 1925; Wolf, 1954; Ehlinger, 1964). Some strains of brook trout and brown trout have been developed to the point where large scale tests indicate a high degree of resistance to the disease. Although furunculosis resistance is a very desirable trait, the resistant fishes seem to have a slower growth rate than less resistant ones (Wolf, 1954; Snieszko, Dunbar and Bullock, 1959). While selective breeding is an effective method of controlling some diseases (Snieszko and Hoffman, 1963), it cannot be relied upon under all conditions.

Acute outbreaks of furunculosis were observed in resistant brook trout when the water temperature was raised by several degrees (Snieszko, 1964). Also poor maintenance and crowding may lower resistance of trout to furunculosis (Kingsbury, 1961).

*Immunization.* Several aspects of the immunization of trout against *A. salmonicida* have been examined by fishery workers. The injection of formalin killed bacterial cells and mineral oil adjuvant produced persistent titers of agglutinins (Reddecliff, 1960; Krantz, Reddecliff and Heist, 1963). Antibody formation takes longer in trouts than in warmblooded animals with maximum titers being reached in brook and brown trouts after three months at 11°C, with a single injection of antigen-adjuvant (Krantz *et al.*, 1963). Once antibody is formed, however, it persists and has been detectable after twenty-four months. The response of trouts to bacterial cells alone is not as good in that lower titers are obtained and antibody disappears within three months (Krantz *et al.*, 1963). Passive immunization of coho salmon (*O. kisutch*) with sera from immunized rainbow trout was successful (Spence, Fryer and Pilcher, 1965) but this is not practical for hatchery use. In fact, the only feasible method of routine immunization of hatchery fishes would be by oral immunization with the antigen incorporated in the feed.

The first attempt at oral immunization (Duff, 1942) using chloroform-killed cells incorporated in the feed was considered a success, however subsequent trials using both living and killed cells gave equivocal results (Snieszko and Friddle, 1949; Krantz *et al.*, 1964). A recently developed technique involving a toxoid, prepared from an endotoxin of *A. salmonicida*, incorporated into pelleted food promises to make oral immunization of trouts against furunculosis practical and effective (Klontz, 1966). Oral administration of the antigen produced specific antibodies which were detectable by immunofluorescence in thirty-four days.

*Prophylactic chemotherapy.* Although the practice of feeding low levels of drugs to control enzootic furunculosis may be useful, it must be done with caution to avoid toxicity to the fishes and alertness to possible appearance of drug resistant strains of *A. salmonicida.* Generally the practice should be avoided since sulfonamide and antibiotic resistant strains of *A. salmonicida* are known to occur.

## Treatment

### HISTORICAL DEVELOPMENT

When all preventive measures for furunculosis control fail, treatment is the only effective means of saving an infected population. Sulfonamide chemotherapy of bacterial fish diseases was initiated in 1937 with the use of 2 grams of sulfanilamide per kilogram of trout per day in an effort to cure brook trout of ulcer disease (Tunison and McKay, 1937). There was no therapeutic effect and some trout died from an apparent toxic effect. Several sulfonamides and a nitrofuran were then tested for their effectiveness in curing 8-month-old brook trout naturally infected with furunculosis (Gutsell, 1946, 1948). Results showed sulfamerazine used at the rate of 17.6 grams per 100 kilograms per day was effective; sulfathiazole at the same rate was less effective, and sulfanilamide and sulfadiazine which followed the nitrofurazone treatments were of little benefit. Nitrofurazone (Furacin) was ineffective when added to the water but was of some benefit when given in food at approximately half the level of the sulfonamides. Further experiments with sulfamerazine showed that daily dose rates of 11, 22, and 33 grams per 100 kilograms continued for forty-five days were not lethal or toxic to brook, brown, or rainbow trout. However growth rates of the trouts varied. Rainbow trout grew normally but growth of brook trout was reduced at the higher level and brown trout growth was stopped by the lowest level because they would not eat the medicated food (Gutsell and Snieszko, 1949a). It was subsequently found that brown trout will eat food containing sulfisoxazole (Gantrisin) at the level of 20 grams per 100 kilograms of trout (Snieszko and Wood, 1955). Sulfamerazine was found to be effective in controlling furunculosis in brook trout at daily levels of 8.8–26.4 grams per 100 kilograms with the recommended level of 17–20 grams per 100 kilograms body weight per day for at least three weeks (Gutsell and Snieszko, 1949b). Treatment of furunculosis infected brook trout with 13.2 grams per 100 kilograms of sulfamerazine or sulfamethazine; 26.4 grams per 100 kilograms of sulfathiazole; or a mixture of sulfamerazine and sulfathiazole again showed sulfamerazine to be most effective, with sulfamethazine second best, and only slight benefit from sulfathiazole or the mixture (Snieszko, Gutsell and Friddle, 1950).

Studies on the tissue levels of the sulfonamides in brook trout given various dosages showed that sulfanilamide was absorbed fastest and produced the highest tissue concentration but was also toxic. Sulfamerazine reached a peak tissue level in four days and sulfamethazine in ten days which may be the reason sulfamerazine is more effective than sulfamethazine. Other sulfonamides were less absorbed and some not at all (Fig. 3) (Snieszko and Friddle, 1951).

Although sulfonamide therapy has been effective, some toxic effects occur. Brood brook trout fed sulfamerazine prophylactically several days a month for two years became sterile. Gross examination of these fish revealed no abnormal pathology but histological examination revealed massive kidney damage similar to the lesions observed in mammals after excessive sulfonamide therapy (Wood, Yasutake and Snieszko, 1955). These investigators showed that no pathology could be demonstrated in fingerling brook, brown, or rainbow trout fed various sulfonamides for up to thirteen weeks

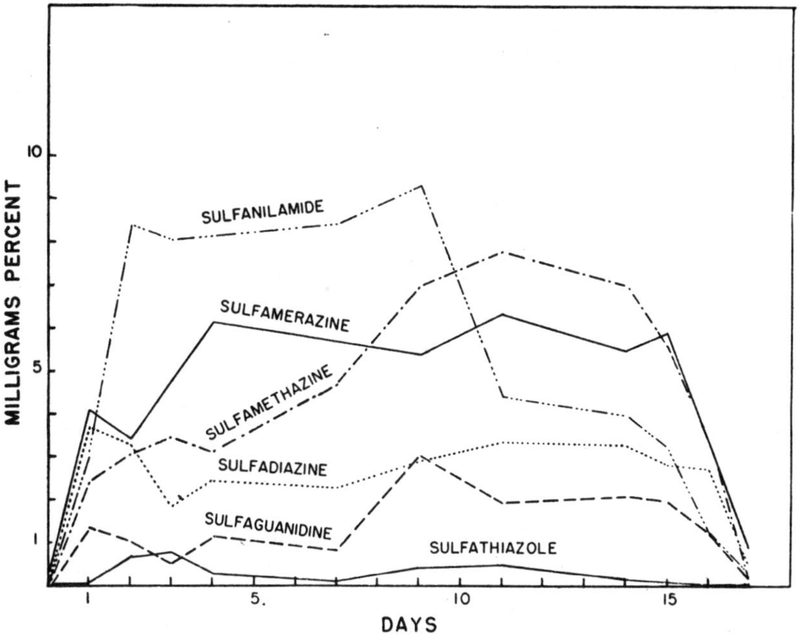


Figure 3. Average tissue levels of various sulfonamides given at a rate of 20 milligrams per 100 grams of fingerling brook trout per day. There was no absorption with sulfathalidine and sulfaquinoxaline. (Snieszko and Friddle, 1951)

but kidney damage similar to that in brood brook fish was seen after twenty-six weeks in fingerling brook trout fed sulfamerazine at 17.6 grams per 100 kilograms either two days a week or one week per month. It was concluded that feeding low levels of sulfa drugs over a long period of time was more harmful than high levels for a short time. Sulfamethazine was considered the cause of an increased mortality of fingerling chinook salmon being treated for a pseudomonad infection, with sulfonamide crystals being observed in histological sections of the kidneys. It was postulated that the salmon may have received too much drug (Wood, Yasutake and Johnson, 1957). To simplify the preparation of food containing sulfonamides, an average dosage of 200 milligrams per kilogram per day or 20 grams per 100 kilograms per day is recommended for routine sulfonamide chemotherapy.

Antibiotics have been found to be useful in treating furunculosis especially if the outbreak is caused by a sulfa resistant strain of *A. salmonicida* which has been isolated from scrapfish such as suckers present in the hatchery water supply (Wood, 1968). Oxytetracycline (Terramycin) and chloramphenicol (Chloromycetin) were found to control furunculosis in adult and fingerling brook trout and fingerling brown trout when given at the rate of 5.0–7.5 grams per 100 kilograms of fish per day for ten to fifteen days (Snieszko, Griffin and Friddle, 1952). Chlortetracycline (Aureomycin) was found to be ineffectual for treating furunculosis in the adult brook trout (Snieszko *et al.*, 1952). However, trout fed chlortetracycline at the rate of 3.8 milligrams per kilogram of trout per day for about two months before spawning had a better survival rate after spawning and about twice the egg hatch of trout not fed the drug (Grassl, 1957). The chlortetracycline was probably beneficial in a prophylactic capacity (Snieszko, 1959).

Although nitrofurazone (Furacin) was one of the first drugs to be tested for use in treating furunculosis (Gutsell, 1946, 1948), most of the experimentation on nitrofurans has been carried out in recent years. Preliminary *in vitro* and *in vivo* experiments using furazolidone (Furoxone, NF-180), nitrofurazone (Furacin), nitrofurantoin (Furadantin), and three other nitrofurans designated as NF-67, NF-23, and NF-86 showed furazolidone to be the best and most of the subsequent work has been done on this drug (Post, 1959). Furazolidone is apparently not very toxic since tests run on a small number of trout showed no apparent toxicity when 5.0 grams per kilogram of trout per day was force fed for fourteen days (Post and Keiss, 1962). Studies have shown that 1.0–7.5 grams per 100 kilograms of fish per day would control furunculosis but the 7.5 grams per 100 kilogram level was best since the disease would recur below this dosage level (Post and Keiss, 1962).

#### RECOMMENDATIONS

Chemotherapy of furunculosis or any bacterial disease should be the last resort in saving the population and should not be substituted for preventive measures. Proper methods of drug-food preparation should be strictly followed and regulations regarding the use of specific drugs for various diseases should be known since these vary from country to country.

#### SULFONAMIDES

Sulfamerazine, sulfamethazine, and sulfisoxazole are the three most widely used sulfonamides. They are used at the rate of 17.6 grams per 100 kilograms of fish per day up to ten days after mortality ceases.

#### ANTIBIOTICS

Chloramphenicol and oxytetracycline are used at a rate of 5.0–7.5 grams per 100 kilograms of fish per day for a total of ten to fifteen days.

#### NITROFURANS

Furazolidone at the rate of 7.5 grams per 100 kilograms of fish per day for ten to fifteen days seems to be very effective. However, more work is needed on dosage levels, toxicity, and tissue residues of this nitrofuran.

# *Septicemic Diseases Caused by Motile Aeromonads and Pseudomonads*

## Introduction

Both warm- and coldwater fishes are subject to diseases caused by water bacteria belonging to the genera *Aeromonas* and *Pseudomonas*. These bacteria are common in freshwater inhabited by fishes and their presence and abundance is related to contents of organic material in water or in bottom sediments. It is not surprising, therefore, that several species of these bacteria have been recognized as pathogens of aquatic coldblooded vertebrates. In marine and estuarine environment, representatives of the genus *Vibrio*, which are taxonomically closely related to *Aeromonas*, were reported as fish pathogens. There is still considerable confusion in regard to types of diseases caused by representatives of these three genera of bacteria. The many names given to these diseases unfortunately were based on some of the symptoms of the particular disease and this has resulted in taxonomically distinct bacteria being implicated in the same disease (redmouth) or taxonomically similar bacteria being involved in differently named afflictions which are probably the same disease (red pest, dropsy, hemorrhagic septicemia). The various names applied to the same or very closely related bacteria also added to the confusion; for example, *A. liquefaciens* has been synonymously known by at least nine different names. While the identification of these aeromonad and pseudomonad organisms is discussed with the particular disease and also in the chapter on identification of fish pathogenic bacteria, most isolates are identified as either *A. liquefaciens*, *P. fluorescens*, or very closely related types.

The best known and economically most important of the diseases attributed to these bacteria occur principally in pondfishes and have been called by several names, of which infectious abdominal dropsy (Bauchwassersucht of European carp) (Schäperclaus, 1954) or hemorrhagic septicemia (Spiczakow, 1933) are the best known.

## Hemorrhagic Septicemia (Infectious Dropsy; Rubella; Redmouth; Red Pest; Freshwater Eel Disease)

### DEFINITION

In the present state of knowledge it is not possible to say with certainty that all the above terms describe one disease with greatly variable symptoms but uniform etiology, or different diseases of uncertain etiology (Otte, 1963; Schäperclaus, 1965). In this text infectious dropsy, hemorrhagic septicemia, red pest, and freshwater eel disease are presented as synonyms for a single bacterial disease caused by *Aeromonas liquefaciens*. Evidence is available showing that hemorrhagic septicemia with symptoms identical to those caused by *A. liquefaciens* can also be caused by *Pseudomonas fluorescens* alone or together with *A. liquefaciens* (Brunner and Striegel-Jaxtheimer, 1951, 1953; Schäperclaus, 1954, 1965). The term rubella is used often in eastern Europe where it is generally accepted that it describes a virus disease of carp which is often complicated with bacterial superinfections. In carp and other pondfishes these infections may occur as: 1) abdominal dropsy in which ascitic fluid accumulates in the distended abdomen; 2) as ulcerative forms in which there are abscesses followed by crater-like lesions in the skin and the musculature; 3) as general bacterial hemorrhagic septicemia. It should be mentioned here that the "red leg" disease of frogs is also caused by *A. liquefaciens*. The term *hemorrhagic septicemia* introduced by Spiczakow (1933) will be used here.

## HISTORICAL

Although the first reports of hemorrhagic septicemia were published by Schäperclaus (1930) the condition was probably common in Europe since the middle ages (Otte, 1963). The disease as described by Schäperclaus was typically characterized by an accumulation of ascitic fluid resulting in a distended body condition and protruded scales (Fig. 4) and it was therefore named a dropsy (Bauchwassersucht).

Figure 4. Roach (*Leuciscus rutilus*) with ascitic form of hermorrhagic septicemia. (Courtesy of Dr. A. J. Timmermans)

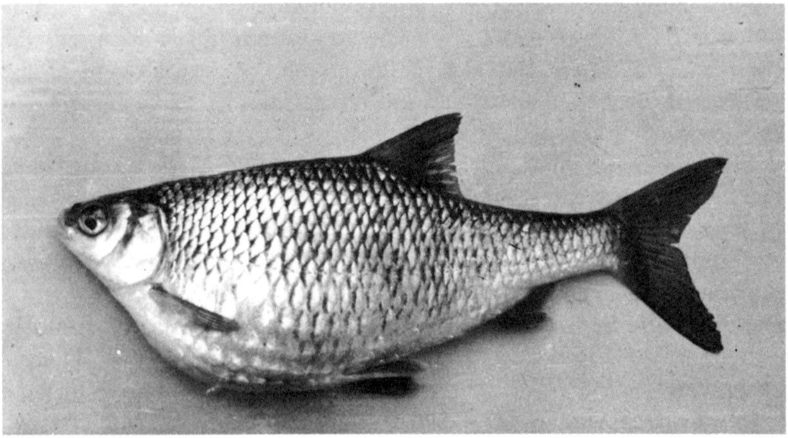

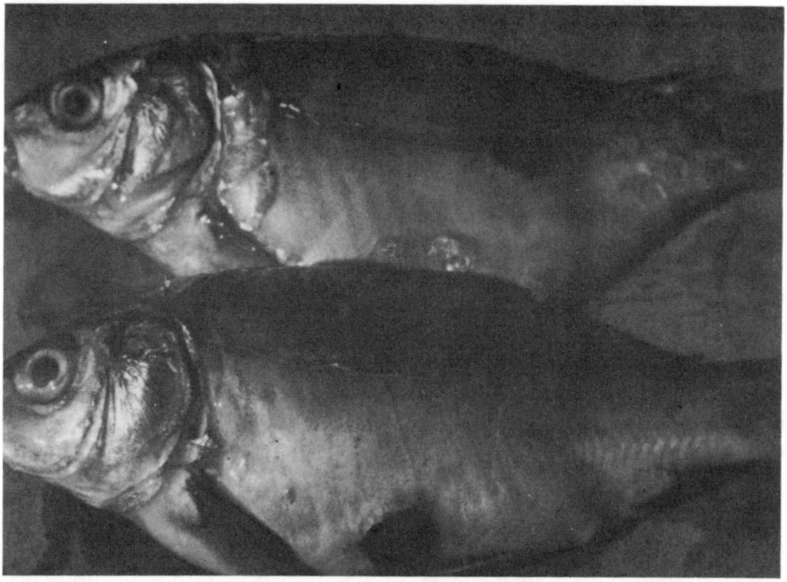

Figure 5. Carp (*Cyprinus carpio*) with ulcerative form of hemorrhagic septicemia. (Courtesy of Dr. Pietro Ghittino.) (This figure, reproduced in color, appears after Index.)

A similar disease was observed in Poland near Lublin in 1924 and was called Lublin disease. In the Polish form of the disease, as differing from the German form, dropsy was infrequent but hyperemia, muscular focal necrosis, deep skin lesions, and general hemorrhagic conditions were recognized as typical symptoms (Fig. 5). Spiczakow (1933) described characteristics of the disease, isolated and identified the causative organism (which was the same as in Germany, *Bacterium punctatum*), and named the disease as hemorrhagic septicemia. Rubella or red pest is characterized by red coloration of the abdomen caused by dermal hyperemia. In the opinion of the Soviet investigators, it is a virus disease but bacteria identified by Soviet microbiologists as *Pseudomonas* and *Achromobacter* are also present (Ljajman, 1949).

SYMPTOMS AND PATHOLOGY

Symptoms of hemorrhagic septicemia have been described by many investigators (Schäperclaus, 1930, 1954; Spiczakow, 1933; Amlacher, 1961) and as with furunculosis several disease forms can occur, of which four can be differentiated (Amlacher, 1961; Otte, 1963).

1. Acute, rapidly fatal septicemia with few gross symptoms.
2. An acute form with dropsy, blisters, abscesses, and scale protrusion.
3. Chronic ulcerous form with furuncles and abscesses.
4. Latent form with no symptoms.

In acute outbreaks of hemorrhagic septicemia there are few, if any, external gross symptoms. Internal congestion of organs, hemorrhagic lower intestine, and petechiae in the peritoneum and musculature may be observed. Such acute outbreaks occur most often in summer within one or two days after fishes are handled or crowded.

Under more natural conditions as exist in ponds the most frequent and extensive epizootics occur in spring during transition from the very cold to warmer water temperature and the stress resulting from overwintering under suboptimal conditions. Dropsical form is most common in carp at that time and results in mortalities within a few days. In dropsical form, clear, yellow, or purulent ascitic accumulations in the abdomen, and degenerative pathology of liver, spleen, kidneys, and of the intestinal tract is often observed. These changes are apparently caused by exo- and endotoxins produced by bacteria. Exophthalmus is common in this form and scales are protruded by the enlargement of the abdomen.

The less rapidly progressing, often chronic form of the disease, is characterized by the appearance of shallow, thin blisters filled with purulent exudate. Such blisters may change to abscesses penetrating into musculature. When these open there are deep, crater-like lesions. Visible dark scars often remain in fishes which recover.

In the latent form, fishes are infected and bacteria can be isolated from internal organs, lumen of the gut, blood, and peritoneum but there are no visible external or internal signs of the disease. Such fishes usually contain antibodies against *A. liquefaciens*.

According to Amlacher (1961), clear separation of the above described forms of the disease is not practical because of the continuous spectrum of transition from one form to another or because of simultaneous existence of dropsical and ulcerative forms. In typical ulcerative form there is no pathological involvement of the liver. In the dropsical form there is advanced

TABLE 3. Hematological data on carp with hemorrhagic septicemia as compared with healthy carp.
After Amlacher (1961) modified.

| *Parameters determined* | *2-year-old carp* | |
|---|---|---|
| | *Diseased* | *Normal* |
| Erythrocytes | 0.73–0.95 $\times 10^6$ per mm$^3$ | 1.5 $\times 10^6$ per mm$^3$ |
| Granulocytes | 90–135 $\times 10^3$ per mm$^3$ | 75–90 $\times 10^3$ per mm$^3$ |
| Ratio of erythrocytes to granulocytes | 8–15:1 | 17–20:1 |
| Differential counts of leucocytes: | | |
| Lymphocytes | 58% | 89% |
| Granulocytes: normal | 12–48% | 11% |
| degenerated | 0–24% | — |
| Hemoglobin g per 100 ml | 2–5.3 | 9.6 |

TABLE 4. Composition of serum of diseased and normal carp. After Amlacher (1961) modified.

| *Component* | *2-year-old carp* | | *Author* |
|---|---|---|---|
| | *Diseased* | *Normal* | |
| Total protein | 0.40–2.75 g % | 1.90–3.95 g % | Dombrowski (1953c) |
| Total protein | 0.30–2.50% | 2.50–2.9% | Flemming (1958) |
| Albumin | 0.07–0.11 g % | 0.86–1.04 g % | ,, |
| Globulin | 0.23–0.49 g % | 1.48–1.98 g % | ,, |
| Uric acid | 0.83–3.10 mg % | 0.56–2.64 mg % | Dombrowski (1953c) |
| Total cholesterol | 15.60–98.0 mg % | 32.60–204.0 mg % | ,, |
| Bilirubin | 0.43–0.85 mg % | 0.13–0.45 mg % | Amlacher (1956) |
| Blood sugar | 14–53 mg % | 40–90 mg % | ,, (1957) |

liver degeneration, toxemia, and disappearance of glycogen. Accumulation of ascitic fluid results from the damage to the liver caused by bacterial toxin. The histopathology of the liver of carp affected with dropsical form of the hemorrhagic septicemia was described in detail (Amlacher, 1961). This author has also reviewed the hematological and chemical changes observed in blood of carp affected by this disease (Tables 3 and 4).

With pondfishes such as golden shiners (*Notemigonus crysoleucas*) in the United States, symptoms may include swellings in the dorso-lateral areas of the body just posterior to the dorsal fin. The swellings may erupt as the disease progresses and form an ulcerous sore. Focal areas of inflammation may also be evident in the kidney (Meyer, 1964). External symptoms in catfish by *A. liquefaciens* consist of large, shallow, necrotic areas on the head (Fig. 6).

### ETIOLOGY

The etiology of hemorrhagic septicemia is still disputed with both bacteria and a virus, together or singularly, being postulated as primary agent(s). The ideas regarding the etiology were reviewed by Schäperclaus (1954, 1965) and most completely by Otte (1963). Readers are referred to these publications for detailed review of references. Otte divided these ideas in three categories. The first idea represented chiefly by German and Polish investigators consider environmental conditions as trigger mechanisms which make fishes susceptible to infection with *Aeromonas* and *Pseudomonas*. The other group represented mainly by Russian investigators, but supported also in Germany and Yugoslavia, considers an unidentified virus as the primary etiologic agent. The third group, consisting of some German, Polish, and American investigators, consider *A. liquefaciens* as the agent of this disease. A disease with so far indistinguishable symptoms can also be caused by *P. fluorescens*. The role of environmental conditions is believed to be of primary importance.

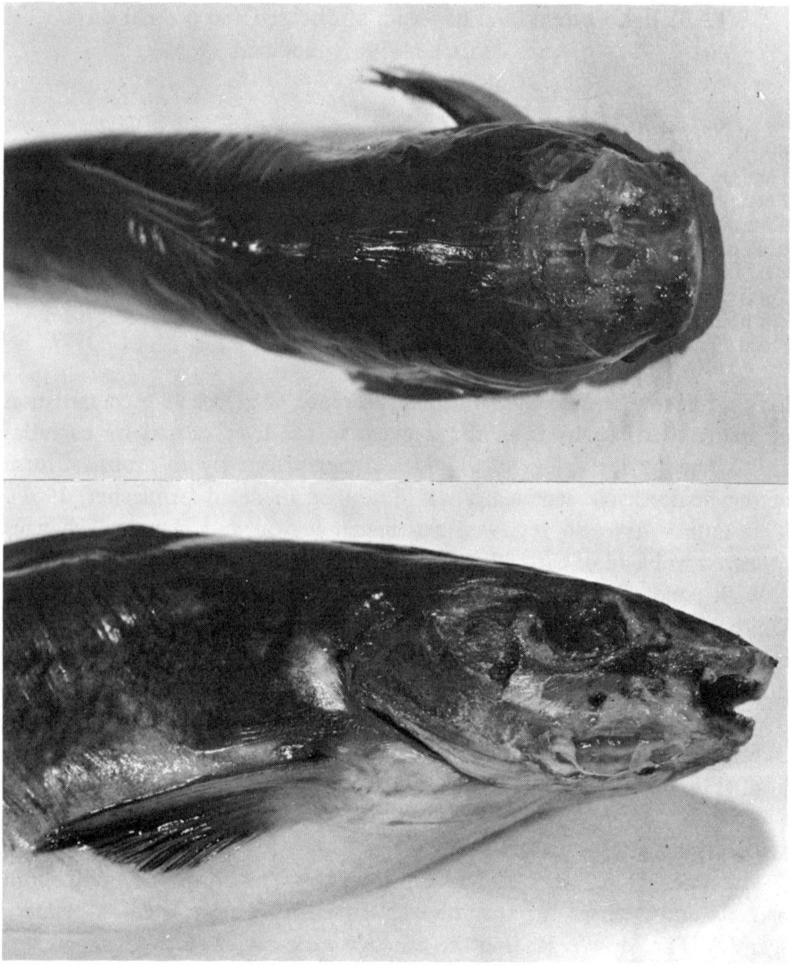

Figure 6. Channel catfish (*Ictalurus punctatus*) with advanced *A. liquefaciens* infection. Note exposure of muscle and bone in heart area, blindness, absence of barbels, and involvement of opercula. (Courtesy of L. F. Rock)

Reasons for originally considering the disease to be an uncomplicated bacteriemia were recently restated by Schäperclaus (1965). He had observed that *A. punctata* was present in large numbers in diseased fishes and would produce typical disease when injected into healthy fishes. Also antibodies against *A. punctata* were found in carp after natural outbreaks of hemorrhagic septicemia and inoculations of carp with polyvalent vaccine prepared from *A. punctata* resulted in reductions in dropsy victims. Treatment of the disease with antibiotics was completely successful. Thus it seemed that *A. punctata* was the cause of the disease, although *P. fluorescens* (*P. granulata*) alone or with *A. liquefaciens* was at times isolated from carp with hemorrhagic septicemia (Brunner and Striegel-Jaxtheimer, 1951, 1953; Schäperclaus, 1965). These two bacterial species are both gram negative, asporogenous rods which are motile by means of polar flagella. The major difference is that *A. liquefaciens* ferments carbohydrates while *P. fluorescens* oxidizes them, and usually produces a fluorescent pigment. While the taxonomy of *P. fluorescens* has remained relatively unchanged, the same has not been true of *A. liquefaciens*. This bacterium was described under the following synonyms:

*Aeromonas hydrophila*
*Aeromonas punctata*
*Bacillus punctatus*
*Bacillus ranicida*
*Bacterium punctatum*
*Proteus hydrophilus*
*Pseudomonas granulata*
*Pseudomonas hirudinis*
*Pseudomonas punctata*

Schäperclaus (1930) has termed the strongly pathogenic strains as *P. punctata* forma *ascitae* and the less virulent strains as *P. punctata* forma *typica*. The former was supposed to cause the dropsical and the latter the ulcerative form of the disease.

Although he later questioned the viral etiology, Schäperclaus (1939) attempted to transmit hemorrhagic septicemia, with partial success, by injecting material which had been filtered to remove bacteria. He attributed the resulting pathology to bacterial toxin. The supporting evidence presented by Soviet investigators for the viral etiology of rubella was reviewed by Otte (1963) and by Goncharov (1959, 1965). These observations showed that carp were infected with bacteria-free filtrates from hemorrhagic skin lesions, with resulting production of exudate and inflammation; that Epshtain-Peshkov inclusion bodies were reproduced in infected fish, and that ultrafiltrates from infected carp produced a cytopathogenic effect when inoculated into cultures of heart, kidney, and fin tissues. Specific viral antibodies have been found in sera of fishes which survived hemorrhagic septicemia. Tomašec and Fijan (1965) obtained a filterable agent from hemorrhagic septicemia and passaged it in explant tissue culture but did not identify the implicated virus. The German investigators of the Munich School (Roegner-Aust, Brunner, and Jaxtheimer, 1950; Roegner-Aust, 1953) observed particles recognized as virions in abdominal exudate or ultrafiltrate from soft organs of diseased carp.

There is evidence for both viral and bacterial etiology of hemorrhagic septicemia but unequivocal evidence is lacking for either view. A blending of the two opposing views postulates a synergistic action between a virus and the bacteria (Dombrowski, 1953a). Supporting the combined etiology was the observation that carp were experimentally infected and killed with bacteria alone but no dropsy was observed unless organ filtrates and bacteria were used (Lucky, Mesároš and Pleva, 1962). Resolutions accepted at the Symposium on Diseases of Fish at Munich, Germany in 1965 established hemorrhagic septicemia as an infectious disease probably of viral origin quite frequently associated with bacteria belonging to the family *Pseudomonadaceae* (Ghittino, 1966a).

Three postulations have been made:

1. Disease is caused by a virus, and aquatic bacteria as *A. liquefaciens* or *P. fluorescens* are casual contaminants. This opinion prevails in eastern Europe.
2. Disease is caused by a virus but bacteria infect the diseased fish and are responsible for death. This is accepted by some investigators in central Europe.
3. Disease is caused by *A. liquefaciens*, or less often by *P. fluorescens*. This view is accepted by many fish pathologists in central Europe and in North America. Three attempts to isolate virus from pondfishes with dropsical conditions in the United States using cell culture were unsuccessful (Wolf, 1966).

In any case chemotherapy of bacterial infection is effective in controlling mortalities.

So far as we can interpret the voluminous literature on hemorrhagic septicemia, it seems that in most cases bacterial infections with *A. liquefaciens* and in some cases by *P. fluorescens* cause hemorrhagic septicemia. These bacteria which often are only opportunistic fish pathogens, rarely, if ever, cause diseases in fishes living under optimum conditions. Stresses as handling, temperature changes, oxygen deficiency, parasites, starvation, and malnutrition may render fishes susceptible to infection which may result in a severe disease. It should be stated once more that until a virus is isolated and characterized, we consider hemorrhagic septicemia of carps, also affecting other species of fishes, a bacterial disease caused by *A. liquefaciens*, *P. fluorescens* or both.

#### DIAGNOSIS

Tentative diagnosis may be made on the basis of the gross symptoms: dropsical conditions with distended abdomen, protruding scales, exophthalmus, and presence of ascites in the abdominal cavity. For a definitive diagnosis, isolation and identification of the causative organism is essential.

If one accepts bacterial etiology of the disease, isolation and identification of the pathogen is of the utmost importance. The procedures required for this purpose are described in *Identification of Fish Pathogenic Bacteria.*

If *A. liquefaciens* is present in pure culture, or at least predominant in the lesions, blood, and internal organs as kidney, spleen, liver, or peritoneal cavity of the diseased fish, and if the same organism is found in the vast majority of diseased specimens examined in a population, one is justified in diagnosing the disease as *hemorrhagic septicemia.* On the basis of observations by central European investigators discussed above, isolation of *P. fluorescens* also may be considered diagnostically valid because there seems to be no significant difference between septicemias caused by either of the two bacterial species.

If one assumes that this is a viral disease, isolation of a definite type of a virus would be of diagnostic value. This is still not possible because there is no valid description of the virus which may be etiologically related with this disease.

### TRANSMISSION, EPIZOOTIOLOGY AND PATHOGENESIS

If hemorrhagic septicemia is primarily caused by a virus, with bacteria as secondary pathogens, the mode of transmission is unknown. Since viruses multiply only in living cells, the existence of carrier fishes, or other animals, must be accepted.

If bacterial etiology of the disease is accepted, the reservoir of potential pathogens probably exists in all natural and artificial bodies of water because *A. liquefaciens* and *P. fluorescens* are common freshwater bacteria. Transmission of fish diseases caused by *Aeromonas* and *Pseudomonas* may also occur under normal conditions by external or internal parasites. Büsing (1952) isolated from the leech (*Hirudo officinalis*) an organism which he called *Pseudomonas hirudinis*. This bacterium is identical with *A. liquefaciens* (Snieszko, unpublished). Dombrowski (1953b) isolated *A. liquefaciens* from copepods (*Argulus foliaceus*) and from leeches (*Piscicola geometra*) which were feeding on carp with hemorrhagic septicemia. He also succeeded in transmitting the disease to healthy carp with infected copepods and leeches. If carp were infected from *Argulus*, the incubation period was 28 days but only 12 days if leeches were the source of infection.

Lewis and Bender (1961) transmitted infection to golden shiners (*Notemigonus crysoleucas*) from water containing about 1000 cells of *A. liquefaciens* per ml, if several scales were removed. Incubation period was twelve hours and mortalities ranged from 40 to 60%. Crowding, tumbling, and rough handling contributed also to infection.

It is well known that *A. liquefaciens* is the etiologic agent of the red-leg disease in frogs. Since frogs and fishes in the same area are often simultaneously infected with this organism, it seems likely that in some instances infection may be transmitted from or by frogs. Typical hemorrhagic septicemia was repeatedly reproduced by contact with bacteria in golden shiners by *A. liquefaciens* (Meyer, 1964). The fact that severe outbreaks of hemorrhagic septicemia occur only at certain times indicates that specific conditions must be present to increase the susceptibility of fishes to infection, or to render bacteria more virulent. Schäperclaus (1954) described two forms of *A. liquefaciens*. One called forma *ascitae* is more virulent and causes the dropsical form of the disease while the forma *sacroviensis* is less virulent and causes the ulcerative form of the disease. Other differences between these two forms are as follows:

| *P. punctata* (f. *ascitae*) | *P. punctata* (f. *sacroviensis*) |
|---|---|
| Smooth convex colonies (smooth) | Colonies irregular (rough) |
| Fast liquefaction of gelatine | Slower liquefaction |
| Fast $H_2S$ production | Slower $H_2S$ production |
| Occasional fermentation of lactose | Lactose not fermented |
| Acid and gas from arabinose | Arabinose not fermented |
| Growth at 39°C | No growth at 39°C |

On the basis of this information one would expect *P. p.* forma *sacroviensis* to be less pathogenic because it appears to be a (R) rough form of the organism. One could also reverse the interpretation and say that in early spring when the forma *ascita* of the disease is present carp are more susceptible. The occurrence of forma *sacroviensis* of the disease in late spring or early summer, and gradual shifting from the high incidence of forma *ascitae* to forma *sacroviensis* during the past two decades may be interpreted by increased resistance of carp to this disease. In the United States septicemias in pond-fishes caused by *A. liquefaciens* are often explosive without symptoms of dropsy or ulceration with incubation time of one or two days and very high mortalities occurring within several days (Lewis and Bender, 1960, 1961; Meyer, 1964), The existence of a delicate balance between host and pathogen was well-illustrated by Schäperclaus (1954). He observed that if there are two carp farms, A and B, each with a mild form of hemorrhagic septicemia, transfer of some carp from A to B would result in increased losses of carp A and B in farm B because carp in farm A are not in immunological balance with bacteria present in farm B and carp in farm B are more susceptible to bacteria transferred with carp from farm A.

Schäperclaus (1954) described two sequences of the progress of hemorrhagic septicemia. They are given here in a somewhat modified form. In the first sequence, infection starts through the intestinal wall weakened by winter starvation. Bacterial toxins and proteolytic enzymes damage the intestinal wall. The muscular wall of the intestine becomes oedematous, semi-transparent, and thin. Excessive mucus filling the gut is eliminated through the anus in the form of mucoid casts. Pathogenic bacteria enter intestinal blood vessels and the lymphatic system. Toxins and bacteria accumulate in the liver causing extensive degeneration of this organ, with the appearance of inflamed foci and necrotic areas. Thromboses appear in the liver and ascites accumulates in the peritoneal cavity. Before the fish dies accumulation of exudates occur in various tissues and under the skin resulting in typical symptoms of blisters, exophthalmus, and protrusion of scales.

The other form of the disease occurs later in the spring and throughout the summer, and is usually caused by an external infection resulting from damage to scales or skin by handling (Lewis and Bender, 1961), leeches (Büsing 1952), or parasitic crustaceans (Heuschmann, 1953) which may contain the etiologic agents in their bodies. Blisters filled with light yellow fluid containing blood cells and bacteria appear in the skin. This is followed by necrotic changes in underlying musculature and results in deep abscesses which may break open to the surface.

In both types of the disease the causative bacteria are eliminated in large numbers into water and this results in the spread of the disease until all susceptible fishes become infected, diseased, and die, or recover.

Fishes which recover may have intestinal adhesions, deformed head, lost eyes, distorted verebral column with scoliosis or lordosis, and dark scars where necrotic ulcers were located. The growth rate is usually considerably reduced in carps which survived the disease.

It has been suggested that at low water temperatures the generation time of bacteria is extended to a point where destruction and reproduction of bacteria are equal and a relatively constant population of bacteria is maintained in the tissues. An increase in the environmental temperature would decrease the bacterial generation time, upset the balance between host and bacterium in favor of the bacterium, overwhelm defense mechanisms, and result in a bacteremia (Post, 1963).

Many investigators reported on the deterioration of health conditions of carps and other warmwater pondfishes during the cold winters of central Europe. Flemming (1958), Liebman, Offhaus and Riedmüller (1960) and Riedmüller (1965) determined in a large number of carps the total serum protein as well as albumin globulin ratio. They found that in carps maintained under poor wintering conditions, or with latent or chronic form of hemorrhagic septicemia the total serum proteins decreased. Serum albumin level dropped first and was followed by a decrease in globulins. With the more rapid decrease of serum albumin, the ratio of albumin to globulin changes. Liebman, Offhaus and Riedmüller (1960) recommended segregation of brood carp on this basis and reported that fish with A/G ratio 0.4 to 0.2 had a much better chance to survive the spring outbreak of hemorrhagic septicemia than carp with A/G ratio between 0.2 to 0.1 or less.

In a very interesting article, Steffens (1964) reviewed the literature on the effect that conditions under which fishes overwinter have on the state of their health and their susceptibility to diseases during the following spring. Ivlev (1955) determined hemoglobin and number of erythrocytes in wild carp under three types of overwintering conditions. In a body of water with average concentration of dissolved oxygen of about 3.7 p.p.m. the hemoglobin level was 11 g% in November, but steadily decreased until it reached 4.3 g% in the middle of March and 8.2 g% by the middle of April. In a body of water containing 2.5 to 2.6 p.p.m. of dissolved oxygen, hemoglobin level was stable at about 10 to 11 g% from the beginning of November to the end of March. In April it dropped to 7.5 g%. In carp overwintering in water deficient in dissolved oxygen (1.8–1.9 p.p.m.), the hemoglobin levels increased from November to the beginning of March from 10.7 to 12.8 g%. For about a month from the middle of March, it dropped abruptly to 0.8 to 1.4 g%. Erythrocyte numbers followed closely the changes in hemoglobin levels. Data presented by Ivlev show that when there was adequate dissolved oxygen and favorable overwintering conditions, quantities of hemoglobin and erythrocytes adjusted themselves to the metabolic requirements of carp. When somewhat less dissolved oxygen was available the fish had to compensate by increasing the levels of both. When less dissolved oxygen was available, fish still were able to make compensatory adjustments. Under conditions of prolonged oxygen deficiency (1.8–1.9 p.p.m.), carp at first were able to compensate by increasing the levels of hemoglobin and red cells, but this ability showed a precipitous breakdown early in March. This was followed by a sudden appearance of anemia. Similar conditions of low oxygen caused stress among American shad (*Alosa sapidissima*) and threadfin shad (*Dorosoma petenese*) and brought on an *A. liquefaciens* epizootic in these fishes (Haley, Davis and Hyde, 1967).

Sorvatchev (1957) reported that protein content of carp serum was about one-third lower in March than during the fall and also that the ratio of different fractions of globulins and serum albumins were changing during the winter period (Tables 5 and 6). All this helps to explain why carp are often in a debilitated condition at the end of winter and are more susceptible to infectious diseases. It also shows the value of the work of Liebmann *et al.* (1960) in using the A/G ratio as a measure of the health of carp.

From this brief review, one can judge the importance of environmental conditions in triggering outbreaks of hemorrhagic septicemia.

It is now generally accepted that the nature of pathogenesis caused by all gram-negative bacteria is similar. The disease process is caused by endotoxins which are complexes of protein, lipid, and polysaccharide present in the bacteria cell wall and are released by autolysis of dead bacterial cells (Braude, 1964; Nowotny, 1969). Endotoxins are believed to produce the same general symptoms regardless of the species of gram-negative bacterium from which they are obtained. It seems likely that the disease symptoms and pathogenesis depend more on the species, age, and susceptibility of the host fish and on environmental conditions than the species of the pathogen. Therefore, diseases caused by *Pseudomonas* and *Aeromonas* are very similar and their identification depends on the identification of the pathogen. However in addition to endotoxins, other factors contribute to the pathogenic nature of some fish pathogenic bacteria such as in the case of *P. fluorescens* isolated from rainbow trout with skin lesions. Experiments showed that the pathogenic effect of this bacterium was due to the production of an extracellular proteinase, and that the production of the enzyme and hence the virulence of the bacterium was dependent upon the composition of the growth medium and temperature at which the pseudomonad was grown (Li and Fleming, 1967).

TABLE 5. Composition of muscle and serum protein in fasting yearling carp. (Sorvachev, 1957) (Modified)

| *Date of analysis* | *Serum protein %* | *Total nitrogen per 100 g fresh muscle %* |
|---|---|---|
| | Fish from winter pond | |
| October 20, 1955 | 3.8–4.0 | 2.8 |
| December 24, 1955 | 3.7–3.8 | 2.7 |
| March 1, 1956 | 2.7–2.8 | 2.4 |
| | Fish fasting 3 months in aquarium at 12–15°C | |
| March 15, 1956 | 1.98–2.0 | 1.65–1.69 |
| | Fish from aquarium after 3 months of fasting followed by 6 months of feeding at 12–15°C | |
| November 20, 1956 | 3·72–3.84 | 2.29 |

TABLE 6. Protein fractions in serum of starving yearling carp determined by paper electrophoresis. (Sorvachev, 1957).

| *Serum fractions* | *Before starvation* | *Six month starvation in winter pond* | *Three month starvation in winter pond and 3 months in aquarium* | *Six month starvation followed by 6 months feeding* |
|---|---|---|---|---|
| Total | % | % | % | % |
| Serum protein | 3.84 | 2.73 | 2.0 | 3.72 |
| alpha-globulin | 9.6 | 24.5 | 57.4 | 24.8 |
| beta-globulin | 24.6 | 34.2 | 18.3 | 28.9 |
| gamma-globulin | 43.8 | 26.3 | 16.6 | 30.7 |
| Albumin | 22.0 | 15.0 | 7.7 | 15.6 |

HOST AND GEOGRAPHIC RANGE

Hemorrhagic septicemia is principally a disease of carps and other cultured pondfishes and is worldwide in its occurrence. In addition to eels and European pondfishes, other affected species include: golden shiners (*Notemigonus crysoleucas*), (Lewis and Bender, 1960); channel catfish (*Ictalurus punctatus*); gizzard shad (*Dorosoma cepedium*) (Rock and Nelson, 1965); bream (*Abramis brama*) (Goncharov, 1965), and other warmwater species. The disease also occurs in species of aquarium fishes (van Duijn, 1967; Axelrod, 1962) and salmonids, particularly trout. Dropsical conditions in trout infected with *A. liquefaciens* have been described by Heuschmann (1952) but this is uncommon.

CONTROL

Essentially the same methods of prevention and chemotherapy as discussed under furunculosis can be applied to hemorrhagic septicemia. As always, the preventive measures are the most desirable with treatment reserved when prevention fails.

1. *Sanitation and environmental conditions*

Hemorrhagic septicemia usually occurs in ponds containing much organic matter and fish parasites (protozoan, copepods, leeches, and acanthocephalans) which may aid in spreading disease. It is important to maintain sanitary conditions in ponds by periodic drying and disinfection. A uniform scattering of quicklime or calcium cyanamide at the rate of 4.45 tons per acre has been recommended to destroy *Pseudomonas-Aeromonas* bacteria in the surface layers (3 cm deep) of ponds (Mattheis, 1966). Stocking of disinfected ponds should be done only with healthy fishes from well-managed establishments. The long-established practice of handling pondfishes in the spring when they are weakest and most susceptible to disease is being replaced by overwintering carp in nursery ponds, and moving them when the temperature rises in late spring. Also carp in different nursery ponds are never mixed. A comparison of the two handling methods showed a 42% mortality in carp moved in the fall and handled in early spring, and a 10% mortality in carp overwintered in nursery ponds and not moved until late spring (Rychlicki and Zarnecki, 1957).

For hatchery-reared salmonids, or warmwater and aquarium and other fishes, good sanitation practices and avoidance of overcrowding, low oxygen, and other poor environmental conditions are the best methods of prevention. For example, as mentioned earlier, low dissolved oxygen was postulated as the predisposing environmental stress condition leading to an *A. liquefaciens* infection in American and threadfin shad (Haley, Davis and Hyde, 1967).

2. *Selection for disease resistance and immunization*

There is adequate information showing that incidence of hemorrhagic septicemia is related to non-specific general resistance and specific immunity.

The general resistance was discussed in the section on transmission and only immunization will be discussed here.

Schäperclaus and Mann (1939) observed that carp which survived the spring epizootic developed specific antibodies which were present in the serum until fall. New infection the next spring resulted in reappearance of antibodies of even higher titer than during the previous year. In a large carp population, Schäperclaus (1954) found that early in March 100% of fish were infected, in May 22%, and none were found to be infected in November.

Snieszko, Piotrowska, Kocylowski and Marek (1938) found that on the basis of agglutination and complement fixation tests, *A. liquefaciens* is immunologically very heterogeneous. Very few cultures gave positive cross reactions. Schäperclaus (1954) found that this immunological heterogeneity is of great importance in stocking carp ponds. When carp from two wintering ponds were transferred to separate summer ponds, the incidence of infectious dropsy was not as great as when each summer pond received a mixed population from several winter ponds. The carp population in each winter pond was infected but developed some degree of immunity to the homologous strain of the infective agent but not to the strain present in the fish from the other ponds.

For several years Schäperclaus (1954) experimented with active immunization of carp against hemorrhagic septicemia, using killed and living cultures of bacteria. In the tests carried out from 1936 to 1951 the average losses of immunized yearling carp were 7.3% and in non-immunized carp 22.2%.

Much better results were obtained by Schäperclaus (1954) when, for breeding purposes, carp were selected which survived natural epizootics followed by an artificial challenge with the pathogens. In tests performed between 1937 and 1942, losses among carp from non-selected adults were 60% (5 tests) and in selected resistant carp only 10% (3 tests).

Large scale immunization of carp against *A. liquefaciens* has not been practicable perhaps because of the serological heterogeneity of the strains (Snieszko *et al.*, 1938; Chodyniecki, 1965; Bullock, 1966), or perhaps because there was no concurrent protection against a virus participating in the disease.

In light of the results of Caselitz's (1966) work on the antigenic properties of *A. liquefaciens*, Schäperclaus (1967) renewed investigations on immunization of carp against hemorrhagic septicemia with a new type of antigen consisting of a mixture of soluble and cellular components of one selected strain of this bacterium. Antigen injected with and without adjuvants gave good protection against a challenge with the homologous strain of the pathogen. When the same antigen was used for immunization of fish in ponds exposed to natural infection, the results were unsatisfactory. Schäperclaus is planning further investigations along these lines. Although resistance or immunity can be established at a particular fish farm, transfer of carp from one farm to another can result in an epizootic of hemorrhagic septicemia, presumably because of exposure to a different bacterial strain. The most complete study of the immune response of fish to *A. liquefaciens* was done with trout (Post, 1963). Intraperitoneal injection of antigen-adjuvant gave protection when the trout were challenged, but orally immunized trout had questionable protection when trout were challenged by the homologous strain. Electrophoretic analysis of immune trout serum showed no component equivalent to gamma globulin of higher animals, and specific antibodies were found in fractions which coincided with the alpha and beta globulins of higher animals. The serum proteins containing antibodies were euglobulins, and antibodies were composed of a complex of serum proteins. The matter of identity of globulin fractions in fish and higher vertebrates has not been as yet fully explained.

As compared with non-immune trout the opsonic index was over three times higher in the immune trout (Post, 1963).

3. *Prophylactic chemotherapy*

In a series of reports Schäperclaus (1956, 1958, 1959) described the results of his approach to the prophylactic chemotherapy of hemorrhagic septicemia by means of oral, anal, and intraperitoneal introduction of antibiotics to carp at the time of spring transfer from winter to production ponds. Some of the antibiotics introduced, preferably by intraperitoneal injection, conferred a transient protection against bacterial hemorrhagic septicemia. Such protection lasted from one to two weeks and was usually very effective. Millions of carp are treated in this way every year in central Europe. Of the antibiotics tested by Schäperclaus, the most satisfactory results were obtained with chloramphenicol. Reductions in mortality from 80–90% were obtained by a single intraperitoneal injection of chloramphenicol at 20–50 mg/kg of fish if carp were transferred in early spring. Although this drug works well against *A. liquefaciens*, it is not effective against infection with *P. fluorescens*. Streptomycin injected at the rate of 50–200 mg/kg was more effective against this bacterium (Schäperclaus, 1956, 1958). A mixture of chloramphenicol and streptomycin is also recommended if both *A. liquefaciens* and *P. fluorescens* may be encountered (Schäperclaus and Brauer, 1964).

Carp injected in autumn instead of spring, although showing symptoms of hemorrhagic septicemia, had only a 5.6% loss compared to 54.2% loss in uninjected controls. Also as far as losses are concerned there was no apparent benefit in injecting carp in autumn and spring compared with a single injection in spring. Some benefit was obtained from two prophylactic injections, but not from three. Carp receiving a single injection had losses of 15.5%; those receiving two injections had only a 2.8% loss, and those receiving three injections had a 5.5% loss (Chodyniecki, 1964).

However, prophylactic chemotherapy is not always successful and extensive mortality occurred among a population of carp which had received an injection of antibiotic in the spring. The reason for the mortality was the very long period of cold weather in the spring during which the injected antibiotic disappeared before the water temperature rose and therefore before the carp could build immunity or resistance (Halvelka and Volf, 1965). It was subsequently found that the activity of streptomycin and neomycin, but not chloramphenicol, was increased by acidic condition at a pH of 4.5–5.0 using acetic and oxalic acids (Halvelka and Volf, 1965).

If warmwater or aquarium fishes are held in tanks or shipped in trucks or plastic bags, addition of antibiotics to the water to reduce the load of bacteria may be of definite help in preventing infection from the stress of crowding. Chloramphenicol (Chloromycetin), oxytetracycline (Terramycin) and a mixture of streptomycin and penicillin may be added to the water at the rate of 10–50 mg/liter.

### CHEMOTHERAPY

While drugs are commonly used for prophylactic control of fish infections caused by *A. liquefaciens* and *P. fluorescens*, reports on therapeutic use are relatively scanty. The first use of chloramphenicol for control of disease by *A. liquefaciens* was carried out, not in fish, but in frogs affected with "red-leg" (Smith, 1950). In uncontrolled tests, the author treated frogs by gastric intubation (with 3 to 5 mg of chloramphenicol per 100 g of frogs) twice daily for five days with apparently good results. For the same purpose, Gibbs (1963) used tetracycline hydrochloride at a rate of 5 mg per 30 g of frogs by oral intubation twice a day for six days. Chodyniecki (1965) used levo-rotatory isomer of chloramphenicol mixed with feed and administered to carp at a rate of 30 milligrams per kilogram per day in four dosages once every two weeks, but without any prophylactic or therapeutic value.

Fijan, Kunst and Tomašec (1967) obtained satisfactory results with oral administration of 10 to 40 milligrams of chloramphenicol and 160 to 320 milligrams of furazolidone per 50 grams of carp repeated for five days. The dosage of furazolidone seems to be excessively high. The most recent and detailed reports on the treatment of *Aeromonas* and *Pseudomonas* infections in pondfishes indicated that an infection with *P. fluorescens* in catfish (*Ictalurus catus*) was completely stopped with an I.P. injection of Kanamycin at a rate of 25 milligrams per kilogram of fish, or feeding oxytetracycline at the rate of 2.5 grams per 100 pounds of fish per day (Meyer and Collar, 1964). Mortalities stopped in four days when golden shiner (*Notemigonus crysoleucas*) in a 40 acre reservoir were treated with oxytetracycline given orally with food at a rate 5.5 milligrams per kilogram of fish per day for ten days. Control fish transferred to a 0.1 acre pond continued to die until only 5% were left alive after ten days. The cost of treatment amounted to 3.4% of the value of fish (Meyer, 1964).

Infections in rainbow trout attributed to *A. liquefaciens* with symptoms of red mouth or abdominal dropsy were apparently controlled by oral administration of sulfamerazine at 200–300 milligrams per kilogram of fish per day (Seaman, 1951). Similarly an outbreak in rainbow trout was also controlled with a mixture of sulfamethazine and sulfathiazole (Wagner and Perkins, 1952). Since there were no controls with the tests performed with rainbow trout, the true effectiveness of the treatment can not be ascertained. Antibiotics as chloramphenicol and oxytetracycline administered orally at a rate of about 50 milligrams per kilogram of fish per day for a week to ten days seem to be of considerable therapeutic value.

## Other Diseases Caused by *Aeromonas* and *Pseudomonas*

### AEROMONAS DISEASES

In addition to hemorrhagic septicemia, there are a number of other similar diseases which are attributed to *A. liquefaciens*. In the freshwater eel disease, also known as "red disease," parts of the eel's body show reddening and progressively enlarging ulcers may develop in the skin and muscle (Amlacher, 1961).

Blotch disease has been observed in several species of freshwater fishes, particularly pike, white fish (*Coregonus maraena*), cyprinids, and percids (Amlacher, 1961). A variant of *A. liquefaciens* appears to be the most important cause but *P. fluorescens* and *Proteus vulgaris* have also been considered as causes.

The disease occurs in spring and early summer and blotches form on the skin from loss of scales and destruction of the dermis to the point where the musculature lies free and is surrounded by a white ring of necrotic dermis. Pike also develop muscle necrosis around the eye and gill regions. The lesion slowly spreads over the entire body. Hyperemia of internal organs may develop with the severity dependent upon the species affected (Amlacher, 1961).

Tail rot and fin rot in goldfish were shown to be caused by an organism closely resembling *A. liquefaciens* (Conroy, 1961a). Tail and fin rot will be discussed more fully in a later section.

Two diseases originally described as being caused by *A. liquefaciens* need clarification. The red sore disease of pike (Reed and Toner, 1941) was originally described as a disease caused by *A. liquefaciens*. However, reexamination of the isolated bacterium has shown it to be *Aerobacter cloacae* (Clement and Gibbons, 1960) so that the disease originally described would be one caused by *A. clocae*. Another example is "redmouth" disease which has been described in trout (Seaman, 1951). A disease with similar symptoms was observed in aquarium fishes (Nigrelli, Jakowska and Baker, 1957). While there is little doubt that *A. liquefaciens* is implicated in redmouth in trout, the disease in western United States is caused by an enteric bacterium as yet unnamed (Ross, Rucker and Ewing, 1966). The situation with redmouth is only one of many examples wherein the disease was named according to the symptoms, resulting in confusion in the exact etiology. Also the disease known as "pike pest" has had several different bacteria implicated as causative agents.

The aeromonad disease of yellow perch (*Perca flavescens*) (Ross, Nordstrom, Bailey and Heaton, 1960) was an interesting account of a disease selective for these fish. Several species of fishes, including yellow perch, were experimentally exposed to the bacterium by adding cultures to aquarium water. Only yellow perch became diseased and died and the bacterium was isolated from the kidneys. No bacteria could be isolated from kidneys of any other species. It should be pointed out that although the bacterium from the yellow perch was originally described as belonging to the genus *Pseudomonas*, it is now considered an aeromonad.

PSEUDOMONAS DISEASES

Many fishery workers have described pseudomonad infections in warmwater, coldwater, aquarium, and marine fishes. A study of the characteristics of the fish pathogenic pseudomonads indicate most infections are caused by *P. fluorescens* or very closely related species (Bullock, Snieszko, and Dunbar, 1965). In 1924 a pseudomonad infection was described in mirror and leather carps (Plehn, 1924) and a secondary infection of fishhook wounds in eels was attributed to *P. fluorescens* (Schäperclaus, 1926).

Pseudomonad diseases in salmonids are not uncommon with an air bladder disease reported in young trout (Wolf, 1937), a disease outbreak in salmon (Rucker, Earp and Ordal, 1954), and most recently a detailed description was given of a pseudomonad infection in trout (Li and Fleming, 1967). The pseudomonad closely resembled *P. fluorescens* and was isolated from skin lesions of rainbow trout. Subcutaneous injection of the bacterium into healthy trout caused the formation of large necrotic swollen areas filled with fluid. Interestingly, a typical red leg condition was noted when the pseudomonad was subcutaneously injected into healthy leopard frogs (*Rana pipiens*). The pathogenic effect observed was apparently caused by an extracellular bacterial proteinase.

A case of tail rot in goldfish was attributed to a bacterium whose characteristics suggested it was a pseudomonad (Conroy, 1963a). When the bacterium was injected into healthy goldfish, petechiae and red spots developed on the fins. Poor environmental conditions such as insufficient food and overcrowding were considered as predisposing factors leading to infection. An epizootic among artificially propagated goldfish was apparently

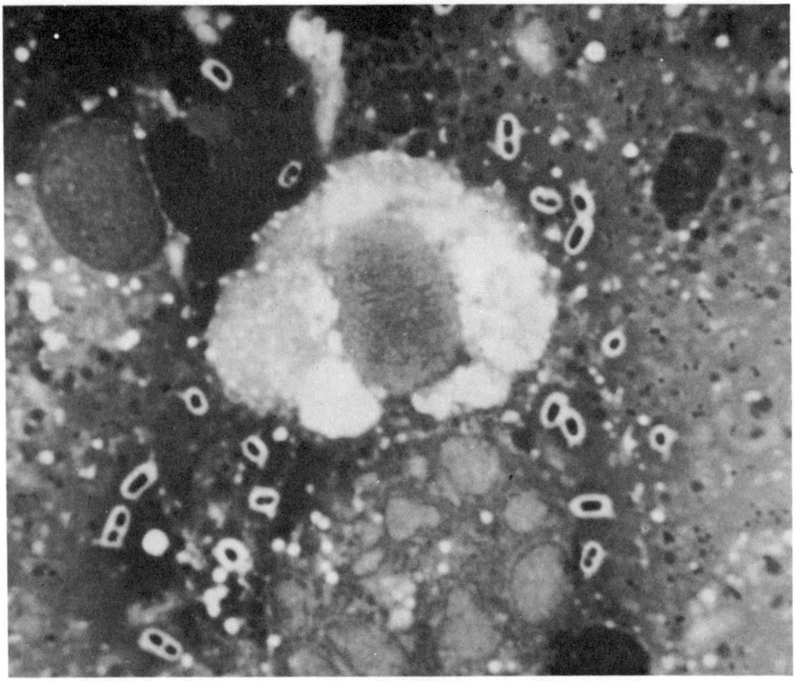

Figure 7. Stained smear from peritoneal fluid of an infected goldfish (*Carassius auratus*) showing the capsulated Pseudomonad. ×1500 (Bullock, 1965b)

caused by a non-motile, capsulated, pseudomonad (Bullock, 1965b). Sick fish exhibited listlessness, hemorrhages on the fins, skin and viscera, and accumulation of bloody peritoneal fluid. When smears from infected fish were stained, the organism was found to have a capsule (Fig. 7) and mucoid growth was apparent on an agar medium. Rainbow trout were killed by peritoneal injection of the organism. Also removal of a few scales from healthy goldfish and adding the bacterium to aquarium water resulted in infection and death of seven out of ten test goldfish. A fluorescent pseudomonad isolated from moribund white catfish (*I. catus*) produced experimental infections in golden shiners, goldfish, and channel catfish (Meyer and Collar 1964). Among the aquarium fishes, epizootics in labyrinth fishes, principally *Trichogaster trichopterus* and *Colisa* species gouramis and paradise fish (*Macropodus opercularis*) were caused by *P. fluorescens* (van Duijn, 1967). Kubota and Kakakuwa (1963) observed the occurrence of an infectious dermatitis caused by *Pseudomonas* spp., which constituted an important cause of loss in marine fish farming operations. The infection was characterized principally by an inflammation and change of color of the skin.

Infections by fluorescent pseudomonads follow the same general pattern as those caused by *A. liquefaciens* in that poor environmental conditions are predisposing factors and in many infections the general external symptoms and internal pathology are very similar, with petechiae and a bloody discharge from the vent being quite common. Thus little can be gained from observing gross symptoms in regard to diagnosis. Accurate identification of the infecting bacterium is the only reliable method of diagnosis.

Unlike furunculosis, which is caused by a single type of a well-described bacterium, the aeromonad and pseudomonad diseases represent many variously named diseases of both coldwater and warmwater marine and aquarium fishes. Since the gross symptoms produced by these bacteria are very nearly the same in most of these diseases, it may be that all these conditions could be grouped under one name, for example, hemorrhagic septicemia of fishes, at least until detailed study of the microscopic pathological changes caused by these bacteria can be determined for each differently named disease. In this way one may see whether or not the pathology is identical in the various diseases or merely superficially the same.

In closing it should be noted that *A. liquefaciens* has been reported to be pathogenic for both warm- and coldblooded vertebrates. Its occurrence as the cause of red-leg in frogs is well known but it also causes ulcerative stomatitis in snakes (Page, 1961) and is becoming recognized as a cause of enteric, urinary, and systemic infections in human beings (Rosner, 1964; Gilardi, 1967; Caselitz, 1966; von Gravenitz and Mensch, 1968).

# *Vibrio Diseases*

## Definition of the Disease

Vibrios are as important as pathogens of marine and estuarine fishes as *A. liquefaciens* is to freshwater fishes, although at times vibrio diseases of freshwater fishes occur such as the recent *Vibrio anguillarum* outbreak in rainbow trout (Ross, Martin and Bressler, 1968). The best known vibrio disease is found in migrating eels (*Anguilla vulgaris*) in salt or brackish water. Similar vibrio infections occur also in other estuarine, saltwater, and occasionally in freshwater fishes, and all will be discussed together. Some investigators call vibrio disease "salt water furunculosis" (J. Wood, 1968).

## Historical

Red pest or red boil disease of saltwater eels (Bergmann, 1909; Schäperclaus, 1927, 1928, 1954) is a serious and economically important disease occurring during the warmer months in brackish and salt water. Reports of disease outbreaks have been numerous from the Danish, German, Italian, and Swedish coasts and the Baltic and North Seas (Sindermann, 1966). It has also been reported from the Netherlands (Schäperclaus, 1927), Poland (Kocylowski, 1963), and Germany (Schäperclaus, 1934). It is probable the disease has been known and reported as early as 1718 from the Italian coast (Hofer, 1904).

During the years 1925–1927 a serious outbreak of "red boil" occurred in the vicinity of Rugen Island and Stralsund in Germany. This outbreak was studied by Schäperclaus (1927, 1928) who isolated *Vibrio anguillarum* from both eels and pike. The disease made its appearance in the pike immediately following its occurrence among eels. It appeared during the months of April, May, and June, which correspond to the breeding season, and affected some 25% of all pike examined. The first external signs were small petechiae in the mouth region and on the opercula, and at times on the ventral body surface (especially in the cardiac region) immediately anterior to the pectoral fins.

A serious outbreak of a vibrio disease among plaice (*Pleuronectes platessa*) has been described by Bückmann (1952). The infection commenced with the production of a red inflammation which later gave rise to abscesses. The diseased fish lived for some four to ten weeks in aquaria, and 70% of all the plaice examined were either suffering from the disease or had previously suffered from it. The presence of the vibrio was definitely established in 49% of the fish, and the remainder showed typical symptoms of "red boil." This disease is of great importance in some coastal regions of Germany and leads to heavy mortalities. Bückmann mentions the natural occurrence of the disease in one-year old plaice, its existence proved by the microscopical examination of stained smears in 87 out of 177 fish. He further placed great emphasis on the importance of "red boil" in coastal waters, where it has given rise to mass mortalities of young plaice towards the end of the pelagic phase of their life cycle. "Red boil" is of grave economic concern to commercial interests in Europe involved with shipment of live eels for human consumption, and the infection is especially predominant in the late spring and early summer months.

Bagge and Bagge (1956) described an ulcerous disease occurring during 1955 and 1956 among cod from the western Baltic, particularly in the Abenra, Alsfjord, Sandvig, and Flensborg fjord regions. According to these workers the disease is confined principally to the western part of the Baltic, the chief distribution being in waters having a surface salinity ranging between 1.5 and 2‰.

A vibrio infection in plaice characterized by a shallow muscular lesion was described by Hodgkiss and Shewan (1950).

Among the cultured fishes vibrios cause serious losses in pink salmon (*Oncorhynchus gorbuscha*) and chum salmon (*O. keta*), and less severe mortalities in chinook salmon (*O. tshawytscha*) and coho salmon (*O. kisutch*) (Rucker, Earp and Ordal, 1954; Rucker, 1959). A vibrio disease of carp was described in 1927 (David, 1927), however as will be discussed later, there seems doubt whether this outbreak was caused by a typical *Vibrio*. Recently vibrio infections have been reported in rainbow trout (Rucker, 1959; Ross, *et al.*, 1968; Hoshina, 1956) and brown trout (Smith, 1961).

Saltwater fish held in aquaria may also become diseased with vibrios.

The current status of vibrio infection in marine fish in regard to clinical symptoms, pathology, etiology, and prophylactic and therapeutic measures has been briefly reviewed by Anderson and Conroy (1969a).

## Symptoms and Pathology

The gross symptoms displayed by vibrio infected fishes are fairly uniform and in many instances similar to those produced by aeromonads and pseudomonads. However, in severe epizootics in eels the disease course may be so rapid that external symptoms are not present (Amlacher, 1961). Diseased eels may show small petechiae in the mouth region, opercula, and ventral surfaces, and bloody abscesses may develop on the skin and musculature (Schäperclaus, 1927, 1928). In most of the affected fishes, freshwater or saltwater, hyperemia of skin and fins, muscular abscesses, and boils, are common external symptoms (Fig. 8). The vibrio infection in the plaice was

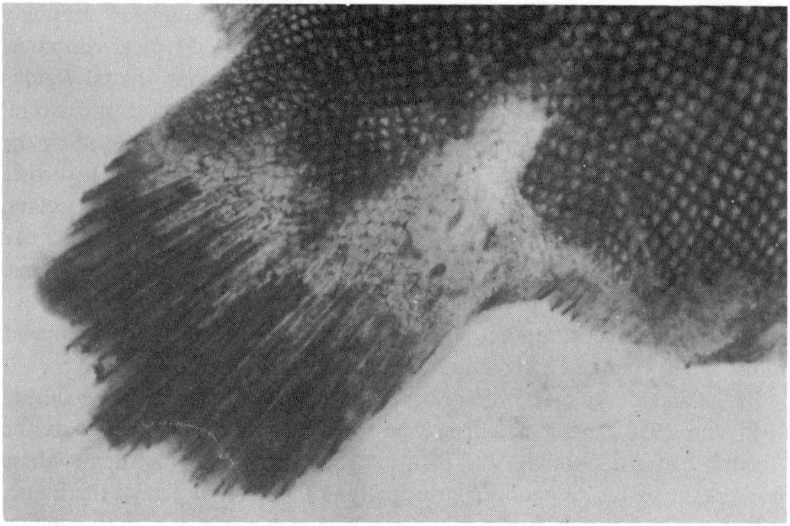

Figure 8. External pathology in Pleuronectidae caused by vibrio infections.
a. Tail rot in Dover sole (*Solea vulgaris*)
b. External lesions in lemon sole (*Pleuronectes microcephalus*).
(Courtesy of Dr. Iain Anderson)
(This figure, reproduced in color, appears after Index.)

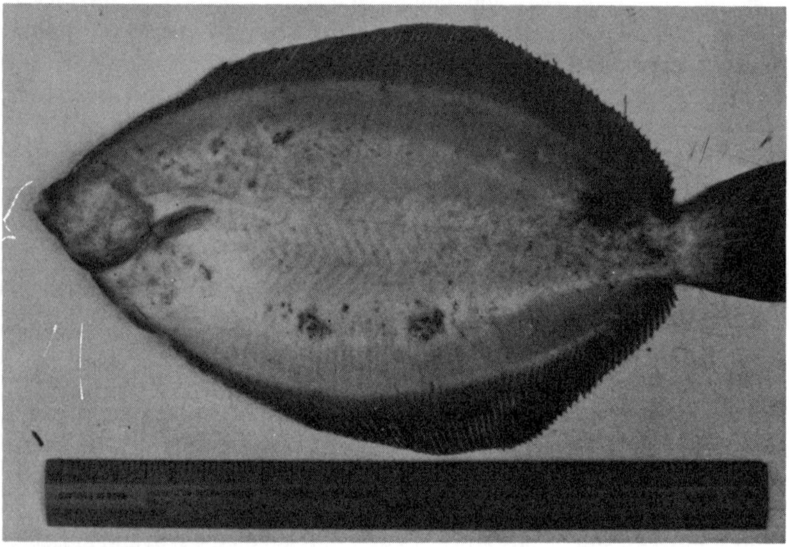

characterized by closed boil-like lesions which were necrotic when cut open (Hodgkiss and Shewan, 1950). Internal symptoms were like the previously described symptoms produced by the other gram-negative bacteria and included petechiae in the body wall, inflamed intestine, swollen and enlarged spleen, and at times swollen and necrotic kidney. Signs of vibrio infection in fishes as reported by many workers have been summarized by Anderson and Conroy (Table 7).

TABLE 7. Symptoms of vibrio disease reported by other workers (Anderson and Conroy, unpublished)

| *Fish species* | *Pathological symptoms* | *Author* |
|---|---|---|
| Cod | Ulceration of body surface, ranging from pin-head sized specks to ulcerative lesions; variation in extent and distribution; sores surrounded by zone of hemorrhage, and covered by grey-yellow necrotic mass; reddish granular tissue or necrotic bone tissue observed underlying ulcers; some sores deep-seated and occasionally fistula-like; no peritonitis observed, although perforation of peritoneal cavity seen on one occasion; ulceration of posterior part of intestinal mucosa present in one individual; complete erosion and ulceration of tail in one case; internal organs apparently normal. | Bagge and Bagge (1956) |
| Finnock, sea trout | No single symptom present in all specimens; congestion of fins; hemorrhage and congestion of anus; hemorrhagic swellings on flank and shoulder; single abrasion of left operculum seen in one fish. | Smith (1961) |
| Rainbow trout | Hemorrhagic or boil-like lesions in body musculature; hemorrhagic ulcers on flank; occasionally exophthalmos; congestion of anus; congestion of liver, intestine and peritoneum; splenomegaly; congestion or necrosis of kidneys; severe anemia in some fish. | Hoshina (1956) |
| | Necrosis and hemorrhage of musculature; inflammation of viscera. | Rucker (1959) |
| Plaice | Inflammation leading to abscesses; osseous tissue frequently affected, particularly opercula; eyes affected, frequently resulting in blindness; inflammatory abscesses of buccal and pharyngeal regions, ventral surface of belly, caudal peduncle, and caudal fin; ulcers of spreading type, commencing as small inflamed area of skin; emaciation. Swollen lesion projected externally from dorsal and ventral surface of body; no apparent damage to skin surface; considerable destruction of adjacent muscle tissue, with necrosis and cavities; swelling filled with pus-like fluid. | Bückmann (1952); Hodgkiss & Shewan (1950); Riddell & Alexander (1912) |
| Yellow-tail, "ayu," wrasse, smelt, horse-mackerel, Pacific mackerel, puffer, "ishidai," file fish | Congestion of dorsal, pectoral, and caudal fins; Extravasation of eye; hemorrhagic lesions and boil-like lesions on body surface and musculature; congestion and dilation of anus; exophthalmos; congestion of intestine and liver; splenomegaly; congestion and necrosis of kidney. Boil-like lesions of skin; hemorrhagic infiltration process; congestion of liver and kidney. | Kubota & Kakakuwa (1963) |

| *Fish species* | *Pathological symptoms* | *Author* |
|---|---|---|
| Killifish, smelt, blenny, goby | Whiteish spot at site of infection, leading to erythema; rapid increase of lesion; dorsal or lateral part of body usually affected; lepidorthosis, sloughing away of scales, necrotic ulceration, and hemorrhage; occasionally exposure of bone; at times perforation of pertioneal cavity, necrosis of muscle tissue, preceding active invasion; "infectious dermatitis." | Zobell & Wells (1934) |
| Chum, pink and chinook salmon | Erythema at base of fins and on lateral sides of body; necrotic zones in musculature; inflammation of intestinal tract. | Earp (quoted by Rucker 1959) |
| Pike | Small petechiae on opercula and mouth region; hemorrhages on body surface leading to bloody abscesses; inflammation of skin; congestion of musculature and jaw; circumscribed petechiae on pectoral fins, jaw, opercula, and thoracic region. | Schäperclaus (1927) |
| | Ecchymosis on body surface; lepidorthosis; localized red spots and blotches on skin and in musculature; congestion of cardiac muscle, gills, and peritoneum; inflammation of lower intestine. | David (1927) |
| Eel | Bloody congestion of fins, particularly anal and pelvic fins; ecchymoses and petechiae on body surface, especially the belly; hemorrhagic ulceration of skin on body, around eyes and mouth, opercula etc., dorsal and caudal fins suffused with blood; frequently detachment of skin in strips; reddening and congestion of anus; marked inflammation of digestive tract; distension of intestine, liver, spleen, stomach, and rectum; congestion of spleen; anemia frequently observed; abscesses may be absent. | Drouin de Bouville (1907) Wolter (1960) |

TABLE 8. Hematological findings on normal and Vibrio-diseased marine fish.
(Anderson and Conroy, 1969a).

| *Fish Species* | *No. examined* | *Hemoglobin gm/100 ml* | *Red cell count* $\times 10^6$ *cmm* | *Hematocrit* % |
|---|---|---|---|---|
| Cod *(Gadus morhua)* | | | | |
| 1) normal | 48 | 6.0 | 1.48 | 25 |
| 2) diseased | 16 | 5.4 | 1.10 | 21 |
| Lemon sole *(Pleuronectes microcephalus* | | | | |
| 1) normal | 12 | 5.5 | 1.39 | 23 |
| 2) diseased | 7 | 4.3 | 0.79 | 16 |
| Plaice *(Pleuronectes platessa)* | | | | |
| 1) normal | 6 | 5.6 | 1.50 | 20 |
| 2) diseased | 4 | 4.2 | 0.78 | 16 |
| Turbot *(Rhombus maximus)* | | | | |
| 1) normal | 3 | 5.7 | 1.45 | 26 |
| 2) diseased | 3 | 4.6 | 0.85 | 19 |

Tissue damage in infected saltwater eels is characterized by dermal hemorrhages in the reddened skin with destruction of the walls of blood vessels allowing extravasation of blood. Hemorrhages are sharply defined in the vicinity of the scale pockets. The walls of the larger vessels in the liver are also destroyed with resulting hyperemia in the areas. Capillary hyperemia is also present (Amlacher, 1961). In pike, inflammation occurs in the hypodermis and sometimes in the muscularis and serosa and between the circular and longitudinal muscle layers. The liver is at times hyperemic and shows coagulation necrosis (Amlacher, 1961). The kidney usually shows no pathology (Amlacher, 1961) but accumulation of pigment with local necrosis of the kidney tubules has been observed (Schäperclaus, 1928).

Anderson and Conroy (1969a) showed that in several species of marine fishes vibrio diseased individuals had a lower red cell count and hemoglobin value than non-diseased fish (Table 8).

## Etiology

A gram-negative, polar flagellated, usually curved rod which ferments carbohydrates and is classified as *Vibrio anguillarum* (or closely related forms) has been isolated from many of the diseased marine fishes, including the eel (Bergmann, 1909; Schäperclaus, 1927; Nybelin, 1935), pike (Schäperclaus, 1928), cod and plaice (Bagge and Bagge, 1956), and several species of salmon (Rucker, Earp and Ordal, 1954; Rucker, 1959). The same organism(s) have been reported from rainbow trout (Rucker, 1959; Ross *et al.*, 1968) and brown trout (Smith, 1961). *Vibrio ichthyodermis** from diseased plaice (Hodgkiss and Shewan, 1950) and *V. piscium* var. *japonicus* from rainbow trout (Hoshina, 1956) also appear to be very similar to *V. anguillarum* (Smith, 1961). The status of *V. piscium* is not clear and since there does not appear to be an authentic culture to work with, the characteristics of this bacterium cannot be redetermined. Although vibrios have been described as curved rods, cell curvature occurs in other closely related genera (*Aeromonas, Pseudomonas*) and taken by itself is of little diagnostic value (Davis and Park, 1962).

The ability to ferment carbohydrates is a recognized characteristic of vibrios (Shewan, Hobbs, and Hodgkiss, 1960a, b) and this is one characteristic *V. piscium* apparently lacks since it has been described as having no action on carbohydrates. Therefore, at this time it is unlikely that *V. piscium* is a true vibrio. Anderson and Conroy (1969a) compared the biochemical reactions of *V. anguillarum* and *V. ichthyodermis* (Table 8a) and concluded that of the more than forty vibrios they isolated from fish some should be biotypes of *V. anguillarum* while others should be classified as

* *V. ichthyodermis* was known as *Achromabacter ichthyodermis* (Wells and Zobell, 1934) and *Pseudomonas ichthyodermis* (Hodgkiss and Shewan, 1950) before being placed in the genus *Vibrio.*

TABLE 8a. Biochemical reactions of biotypes of *Vibrio anguillarum* and of *V. ichthyodermis* (Anderson and Conroy, 1969a).

| | *V. anguillarum* Type A | | | | *V. anguillarum* Type B | *V. anguillarum* Type C | | *V. ichthyodermis* | |
|---|---|---|---|---|---|---|---|---|---|
| | Bagge and Bagge (1956) | Cisar and Fryer (1969) | Muroga and Egusa (1967) | Wolter (1960) | Lagarde and Chakroun (1965) | Smith (1961) | Ross, Martin and Bressler (1968) | Wells and Zobell (1934) | Hodgkiss and Shewan (1950) |
| gelatin liquefaction | + | + | + | + | + | + | (+) | + | + |
| nitrate reduction | ● | + | + | ● | + | + | + | + | + |
| indol formation | + | + | + | + | — | — | — | — | + |
| glucose | A | A | A | A | A | A | A | A | A |
| saccharose | A | A | A | A | — | A | A | A | A |
| mannitol | A | A | A | A | ● | A | A | A | A |
| maltose | A | A | — | A | A | A | A | ● | A |

+ = positive　　— = negative

(+) = weak positive　　● = unknown

biotypes of *V. ichthyodermis*. However. these authors feel that if only a single species of fish pathogenic vibrios is to be used then *Vibrio anguillarum* would have precedence. Most of the fish pathogenic vibrios seem to be similar to or identical with *V. anguillarum*, however serological studies have shown differences among the isolates (Rucker, 1959) and further work is necessary before definite conclusions can be reached regarding speciation. *Vibrio anguillarum* is not recognized in the seventh edition of *Bergey's Manual of Detrminative Bacteriology* (Breed *et al.*, 1957).

It should be noted that although *V. parahemolyticus* is primarily a human pathogen it also causes disease in fishes (Egusa, 1968, per. comm) and the blue crab (*Callinectes sapidus*) (Wang, Colwell, Lovelace and Krantz, 1969).

## Diagnosis

Because of the similarities between *A. liquefaciens* and *V. anguillarum*, not only in the symptoms produced but also the characteristics of the bacteria themselves, the only reliable method of diagnosis of vibrio diseases is by accurate identification of the bacterium. At present this can be difficult and the main diagnostic test is the pteridine agent 0/129 (Shewan, Hodgkiss and Liston, 1954) which inhibits the growth of vibrio but not *A. liquefaciens*. This and other diagnostic tests will be discussed further in *Identification of Fish Pathogenic Bacteria.*

## Transmission and Pathogensis

Transmission of vibrio diseases among saltwater fishes seems to be by fish to fish contact. Since the disease is enzootic in the saltwater eel, this fish may serve as a reservoir of this bacterium. At least one vibrio outbreak among rainbow trout occurred after feeding salmon viscera and marine trash fish which may have contained the vibrio (Rucker, Earp and Ordal, 1954).

At present the mode of pathogenesis of vibrios is not known. It may be assumed that it is the same as with other gram-negative rod-shaped bacteria and caused by an endotoxin.

## Host and Geographic Range

As stated previously, vibrio diseases occur principally in marine and estuarine fishes although important exceptions are the freshwater pike and rainbow trout. Other fishes suceptible to vibrio infections but not previously mentioned include herring (*Clupea pallasi*) (Rucker, 1959), roach (*Rutilis rutilis*) (Schäperclaus, 1934), gurnards (Triglidae), wrasses (Labridae) (Nybelin, 1935), and the queenfish (*Seriphus politus*) (Oppernheimer, 1963). Geographic range appears worldwide. Among salmon the pink and chum salmon are particularly susceptible (J. Wood, 1968).

## Control Measures

### PREVENTION

Immunization, prophylactic chemotherapy, or breeding of resistant strains of fish are technically not practicable as control measures with the saltwater fishes unless cultured or kept in confinement. Several sanitation procedures may help to reduce the incidence of disease. Eels suspected of being diseased should be held in cool fresh water since *V. anguillarum* is a halophilic organism. Such diseased ells should only be held three days at most. The holding and weir areas should be changed often to avoid collection of disease carrying eels which may infect healthy fish. Also the changing of catch areas may reduce incidence of disease. Crowding of holding areas should be avoided and saltwater holding areas should be dried for six months to kill the pathogen (Schäperclaus, 1954; Amlacher, 1961).

Immunization of salmonids has been attempted. Hayashi, Kobayashi, Jamata and Ozaki (1964a) found that a natural immunity against the vibrio disease developed in rainbow trout, but that this acquired immunity was of relatively short duration. Following the oral administration of a concentrated vaccine for four weeks the highest serum titer was 1:128. The weekly injection of the vaccine gave a maximum titer of 1:512, and Hayashi and his colleagues believed that the injection of a concentrated vaccine would prove to be a useful prophylactic measure for the control of vibrio disease in rainbow trout.

### CHEMOTHERAPY

Chemotherapy for disease outbreaks among unconfined marine fishes is not practical as yet. An artificial vibrio infection in rainbow trout was controlled by feeding a diet containing 0.02% furazolidone for two weeks (Hayashi *et al.*, 1964b). A standard sulfamerazine treatment of 8–12 g/100 lb of fish/day has been recommended for vibrio infected hatchery fishes.

Kubota and Hagita (1963) have observed that nitrofurazone was of value in the therapy of vibrio infections in yellow tail (*Seriola quinqueradiata*). The drug was administered orally at a concentration of not more than 56 g/100 kg/day and treatment was not extended over a period longer than four days to avoid undesirable side effects.

In Pacific salmon kept in hatcheries treatment with sulfamethazine and oxytetracycline at the usual rate for ten days is very effective. Prophylactic treatment with sulfamethazine at a rate of 2 grams per 100 lbs per day before the disease appears is also satisfactory (J. Wood, 1968).

# *Redmouth and Other Diseases Caused by Enteric Bacteria*

## Definition of the Disease

The term redmouth as used here will mean the disease of rainbow trout caused by an unnamed enteric bacterium. Original isolations of the redmouth bacterium were made in the state of Idaho in 1950 by Rucker (pers. comm. 1963). Although occasionally seen in other western and northwestern states, the disease occurs mostly in Idaho.

## Symptoms and Pathology

Inflammation and erosion of the jaws and palate in trout is not only characteristic of redmouth, but also occurs in other bacterial diseases such as coldwater disease (Wood and Yasutake, 1956a) and ulcer disease. However, the bacteria responsible for coldwater and ulcer disease are characteristic for their respective diseases and these conditions should not be confused with redmouth. The following symptoms and pathology summarized by Rucker (1966) are often characteristic of rainbow trout with redmouth. The trout first become sluggish and darken in color. This is followed by the characteristic reddening in the mouth, opercula, isthmus, and base of fins. Internal examination of infected trout shows hemorrhages in the body fat and posterior intestine. The stomach may be filled with a watery liquid and the intestine with a yellow fluid (which is characteristic of many gram-negative infections). Histopathological examination of tissues from infected trout show that the disease is an acute bacteriemia with bacteria and the accompanying inflammatory response occurring in virtually all tissues. Bacteria are especially conspicuous in vascular tissue and in the petechial hemorrhagic areas which give the redmouth appearance.

## Etiology

The causative agent of redmouth is a gram-negative, straight or slightly curved rod which is $1.0\mu \times 2.0\text{–}3.0\mu$. The bacterium is peritrichously flagellated and a thorough study of its other cultural and biochemical properties indicates that it belongs in the family Enterobacteriaceae (Ross, Rucker and Ewing, 1966). Although the redmouth bacterium resembles several members of this family in its biochemical and serological reactions it is not identical to any described species and at this time the bacterium has not been classified as to genus and species.

## Diagnosis

Since the described external pathology and symptoms may occur in several bacterial diseases, proper diagnosis of redmouth must be made by isolation of the bacterium and demonstration that it has the same characteristics as the organism described by Ross *et al.* (1966). Since the disease is rather limited in the trout growing areas of Idaho, tentative diagnosis may be made on the basis of symptoms and location of diseased trout.

## Transmission and Pathogenesis

Experimental transmission of redmouth has been accomplished by two methods. In the first, fourteen three- to four-inch rainbow trout which had died from redmouth were placed in a compartment ahead of fifty healthy three- to four-inch rainbow trout from a hatchery free of redmouth. The redmouth organisms were carried from the dead trout in the water to the healthy trout and this resulted in a 52% mortality after nineteen days. In the second method, approximately 500 milliliters per day of a growing broth culture of the redmouth bacterium were dripped into water containing fifty healthy four-inch rainbow trout. The culture was added for four days and after eighteen days, thirteen of the trout had died. In both transmission experiments, pure cultures of the redmouth bacterium were obtained from trout which had died (Rucker, 1966). The most likely means of natural transmission would be by fish to fish contact or exposure of healthy trout to bacteria shed by carrier trout.

The mode of pathogenesis is not known.

## Host and Geographic Range

Redmouth has reportedly occurred only in rainbow trout. Most outbreaks occurred in Idaho but some have occurred in Colorado, Nevada, California, and Arizona (Ross *et al.*, 1966).

## Control

### PREVENTION

In redmouth, as in all communicable diseases, observation of strict sanitary practices and elimination of possible carrier fish from the water supply are extremely important. Oral immunization against redmouth using a killed cell bacterin incorporated into pelleted food has been tested as a means of controlling the disease. To test the efficacy of such a bacterin, fingerling rainbow trout obtained from a hatchery where redmouth had never been diagnosed were fed pelleted food containing 15 grams wet weight of bacterial cells per pound of trout-feed meal. The food containing bacterin was fed five times a week for two weeks and then once a week. Seventy days after immunization procedure had been started, the trout, along with control trout which received no bacterin, were challenged with the redmouth bacterium. Ten immunized and ten control trout were injected intra-peritoneally with a dose calculated to contain one $LD_{90}$ of the redmouth organism. After eleven days there were nine survivors in the orally immunized group and one survivor in the nonimmunized control group. Subsequent challenges of immunized and nonimmunized trout gave similar results and these are summarized in Table 9. The practicability of oral immunization against redmouth has not been tried on a large scale.

CHEMOTHERAPY

Outbreaks of redmouth have been successfully treated by a combination of sulfamerazine and antibiotics. Sulfamerazine at the rate of 20 grams per 100 kg of fish per day was given for five days followed by three days of oxytetracycline or chloramphenicol at 5.0 grams per 100 kg of fish per day (Rucker, 1966).

TABLE 9. Summary of response of immunized and control rainbow trout to challenge doses of virulent redmouth organisms at several time intervals (Ross and Klontz, 1965).

| | *Survivors* | | | |
|---|---|---|---|---|
| *Days* | *Immune* | *Control* | *Dosage* | |
| 70 | 9/10 | 1/10 | 1 $LD_{90}$ | |
| 98 | 10/10 | 4/10 | 1 $LD_{90}$ | |
| 304 | 9/10 | 4/10 | 1 $LD_{90}$ | |
| 339 | 9/9 | 4/10 | 5 $LD_{90}$ | — previous challenge: 304 days |
| | 10/10 | 1/10 | 1 $LD_{90}$ | |
| 360 | 7/10* | 2/10† | 1 $LD_{90}$ | |
| | | 1/10 | 1 $LD_{90}$ | |
| | 11/16 | 0/10 | 40 $LD_{90}$ | |
| 408 | 9/9 | 1/10 | 10 $LD_{90}$ | — previous challenges: 304 and 339 days |
| Total | 45/50 (90%) | 12/60 (20%) | 1 $LD_{90}$ | |
| | 9/9 (100%) | 1/10 (10%) | 10 $LD_{90}$ | |
| | 11/16 (69%) | 0/10 (0%) | 40 $LD_{90}$ | |

* These fish were fed a mixture of redmouth and *A. salmonicida* bacterin.
† These fish were fed *A. salmonicida* bacterin.

## Other Diseases Caused by Enteric Bacteria

Many infections of fish and other poikilotherms have been described as due to *Proteus*, but it is likely that the majority of these organisms would now be considered as pseudomonads or aeromonads.

Babes and Riegler (1903) observed an epizootic among freshwater fishes in Bucharest and other places in Romania from which they isolated an organism described as *Proteus piscicidus versicolor*. A severe epizootic of a so-called "proteobacillosis" has been mentioned by Chiesa (1945) from the River Parana in Argentina. This report is of particular interest as it constitutes one of the earliest records of bacterial fish diseases in that country.

The infected fishes presented symptoms of small tumor-like growths on the ventral parts of the body, posterior to the pectoral fins. Occasionally the same picture was observed on the dorsal body surface and on the head. The affected areas were soft and filled with a purulent fluid. The surrounding skin was of a reddish color, and definitely necrotised. Internally the organs were congested and suffused with blood, while the peritoneal cavity was filled with a bloody serous fluid. The liver and pancreas were especially affected, being totally covered with petechiae. A number of pinkish-colored blotches were observed on the internal surface of the abdominal wall, and the muscular tissue was invaded. From the foregoing description it is possible to note a certain similarity to diseases caused by aeromonads or pseudomonads, in spite of which the disease has been considered in the present chapter under the original definition given as "proteobacillosis."

Hoshina (1962) recently studied an epizootic disease resembling "red pest" in eels, which appears to be quite common in Japan. He found that it may be caused by *Aeromonas punctata*, a paracolon, or a combination of the two. The paracolon was isolated from muscular abscesses, the liver, kidney, blood, and intestinal tract of the diseased eels, and was described by Hoshina as *Paracolobactrum anguillimortiferum*. This organism is a gram-negative, asporogenous, non-encapsulated rod, measuring 0.9–1.6$\mu$ × 0.5–0.8$\mu$. It is motile by means of peritrichous flagella. Experimentally it was shown that the organism is pathogenic to eels, carp, goldfish, rainbow trout, frogs, and mice, following intramuscular and intra-peritoneal injection, but was non-pathogenic to mice when administered *per os*. Hoshina concluded that by virtue of its fermentative attack on glucose and its pathogenicity to fishes, the organism resembled *Aeromonas*. However the possession of peritrichous flagella caused him to note its affinity with *Achromobacter*. Finally he concluded that it was a paracolon, even though it failed to ferment lactose, for which reason it was designated *Paracolobactrum anguillimortiferum*.

# *Ulcer Disease*

## Definition of the Disease

Symptomatically, any fish with external lesions or ulcers can be said to have ulcer disease. Although skin ulcerations are present in many bacterial fish diseases, the term ulcer disease is used here to indicate the bacterial disease of trout, particularly brook trout, caused by *Hemophilus piscium.*

## Historical

On the basis of the description of symptoms, Calkins (1899) reported this disease first. Since protozoans were seen in the infected fish, the disease was thought to be caused by a parasite. The term "ulcer disease" was first used by Marsh in 1905 but was only a general term to describe the external ulcerous condition. Diseases of brook trout with symptoms very similar to those described by Marsh were described in Europe (Hofer, 1904) and again in the United States (Fish, 1934; Wolf, 1939, 1941). Most investigators reported the occurrence of gram-negative bacteria in the lesions, and Fish (1934) isolated twenty-three pure cultures of bacteria from lesions. Of these cultures, twenty-two proved to be non-pathogenic when injected intradermally or subcutaneously into fingerling brook and rainbow trouts. The one culture which was pathogenic was identified as *A. liquefaciens*, a recognized fish pathogen. However Fish was not sure of the role, if any, *A. liquefaciens* played in ulcer disease. Since *A. salmonicida* could also, at times, be isolated from trout with ulcer disease, some workers believed the shallow red lesions were some less-common symptoms of furunculosis and that ulcer disease was another form of furunculosis. Fish (1934) pointed out that the lesions of ulcer disease and furunculosis were quite different and that ulcer disease was more of a localized infection whereas furunculosis was a definite septicemia. The confusion as to the exact nature of ulcer disease was cleared up when it was shown that ulcer disease and furunculosis were two different diseases which often occurred simultaneously in brook trout (Snieszko and Friddle, 1950). When the diseases occurred together, *A. salmonicida* could be isolated easily but the ulcer disease bacterium would not grow on the same medium, except as tiny colonies which developed after three to four days in the blood carried over from inoculation. However, when whole blood or fish peptone (an enzymatic extract of brook trout tissue described in *Identification of Fish Pathogenic Bacteria*) was added to media, the ulcer disease bacterium grew well. When trout free of furunculosis were exposed to pure cultures of the isolated bacterium they displayed the typical ulcers, and the causative agent was reisolated in pure culture thus fulfilling Koch's postulates (Snieszko and Friddle, 1950).

In the late 1940's and early 1950's ulcer disease caused serious mortalities in hatchery brook trout in the eastern United States, often wiping out entire populations of fish (Snieszko, 1952). As previously mentioned, ulcer disease and furunculosis often occurred together and would cause greater mortality than either disease alone. In the last ten years however only a few light outbreaks of ulcer disease have been reported among hatchery trout.

## Symptoms and Pathology

Ulcer disease is characterized by shallow open sores on the body surface (Fig. 9) which occasionally may resemble furunculosis lesions (Davis, 1953). Ulcer disease usually begins as a localized external infection. Affected trout become acutely diseased and die when the infection becomes systemic. Development of the ulcer disease lesion has been described in detail (Wolf, 1939; Fish, 1934) and according to Fish (1934) the earliest lesion to appear on the body is a definite epithelial thickening which produces a small white tuft or patch 0.5–1.0 millimeter in size. The patch loosens from the body surface and may superficially resemble a fungal growth. The white patch has been described as an "epithelial tuft." The tuft gives way to erosion of the skin and the formation of a well defined, circular, shallow, dark red, or gray ulcer. Several ulcers may coalesce to form irregular ulcerated areas. In many outbreaks ulcers may also form on the fins between the rays, or on

Figure 9. Typical ulcers in brook trout (*Salvelinus fontinalis*) with ulcer disease.

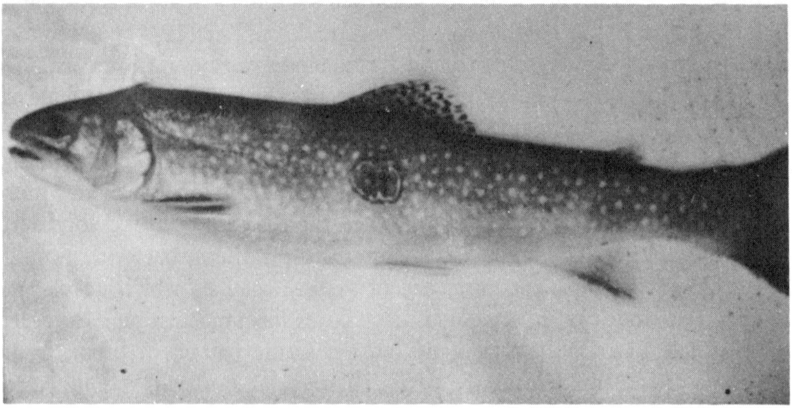

the edges of the jaw or roof of the mouth. The causative bacterium is confined to the dermal lesion and does not invade the body muscle. As the dermis is destroyed the bacteria may be washed out of the lesion (Wolf, 1939; Snieszko, 1952; Davis, 1953). In a few cases of ulcer disease in rainbow trout the ulcer involved the body muscle and was identical in appearance to a furuncle seen in fish furunculosis. In acute ulcer disease in brook trout, typical ulcers may be absent and the gross internal symptoms are the same as in acute furunculosis, and *H. piscium* is present in the tissues and internal organs (Snieszko, 1952). Internal symptoms are present only when the disease becomes systemic and pathological changes grossly resemble those caused by *Aeromonas* and *Pseudomonas* infections.

## Etiology

The causative agent of ulcer disease is a gram-negative non-motile rod which is 0.8μ wide by 1.0–3.0μ long. Its characteristics have been determined and it is presently classified as *Hemophilus piscium* (Snieszko, Griffin and Friddle, 1950). Unlike the other gram-negative fish pathogens, *H. piscium* will not grow on general laboratory media unless diphosphothiamine or adenosine triphosphate are added to the medium (Griffin, 1951). These growth factors may be supplied to the medium in the chemically pure form or as fish peptone. A simplified medium consisting of Mueller Hinton (Difco) medium plus diphosphothiamine has been recently described (Bullock, 1965a).

## Diagnosis

The only positive diagnosis of ulcer disease is by isolation and identification of *H. piscium*. This is described in *Identification of Fish Pathogenic Bacteria*.

## Transmission

When an active infection is present, bacteria are shed from the open lesion and with the fecal material into the water where they may infect other trout. Adult fish surviving the disease may act as carriers. As previously stated, the bacteria gain entrance through the epithelium although it is not known whether they are capable of penetrating the intact epithelium (Davis, 1953). Since the bacterium is nutritionally fastidious it is doubtful that it could survive in water for long periods.

## Host and Geographic Range

So far the disease is limited to salmonids and the eastern brook trout is the most susceptible. However as in furunculosis different strains of brook trout vary in their susceptibility to the disease (Snieszko, Dunbar and Bullock, 1959). Brown and lake trout may become infected. Rainbow trout are more resistant but may become infected and diseased. The disease is reportedly limited to the eastern United States and eastern Canada (Margolis, 1954; Rabb and McDermott, 1961).

## Control

### PREVENTION

Prevention of ulcer disease generally follows the same methods as outlined for the bacterial diseases already discussed. Strict sanitation of hatchery equipment, elimination of carrier fish from the water supply, and raising resistant strains of fish are commonly used methods. It is interesting to note that trout which are resistant to furunculosis are usually also resistant to ulcer disease, possibly because the two diseases often occur together.

### CHEMOTHERAPY

Before the etiology of ulcer disease was known, external disinfectants were used but were of no benefit. Later sulfonamides were tried as chemotherapeutic agents but these too were generally ineffective (Wolf, 1941). However in one instance sulfamerazine fed at a level of 3 grams per pound of feed for twelve to nineteen days was reported to reduce mortalities in trout with ulcer disease (Wolf, 1947). However it must be remembered that at the time of this report *H. piscium* was unknown and it is possible the trout had ulcer disease complicated by furunculosis. In such a mixed infection, sulfamerazine might have controlled furunculosis and reduced mortalities. In controlled experiments by Snieszko, Griffin and Friddle (1952) trout known to be infected with *H. piscium* were treated with oxytetracycline, chlortetracycline or chloramphenicol. Treatment levels varied from 25–75 milligrams per kilogram of fish per day and treatment time lasted up to forty-seven days. Chloramphenicol and oxytetracycline were effective in controlling ulcer disease but chlortetracycline was of no benefit even at the 75 milligram per kilogram level (Fig 10). Since the *in vitro* results showed chlortetracycline to be effective against *H. piscium*, it was assumed the drug was not effectively absorbed from the intestinal tract or was inactivated after absorption. Even though Snieszko and his associates found that 50 milligrams per kilogram of body weight per day of oxytetracycline was an effective dosage for treating ulcer disease, they suggested that the maximum dose of 75 milligrams per kilogram of body weight per day be used to provide a margin of safety, at least during the first several days of treatment. They stressed the importance of beginning treatment as soon as possible after an outbreak of ulcer disease has started and also removing visibly sick fish since they would probably not be saved and would serve as a reservoir of the pathogen. Treatment should last until the epizootic is under control and this may be achieved after ten to fifteen days. It has also been suggested (Snieszko *et al.*, 1952) that a more permanent control of ulcer disease may be achieved by replacing oxytetracycline with chloramphenicol during the last four to six days of treatment. The dose rate for chloramphenicol is the same as for oxytetracycline, namely 75

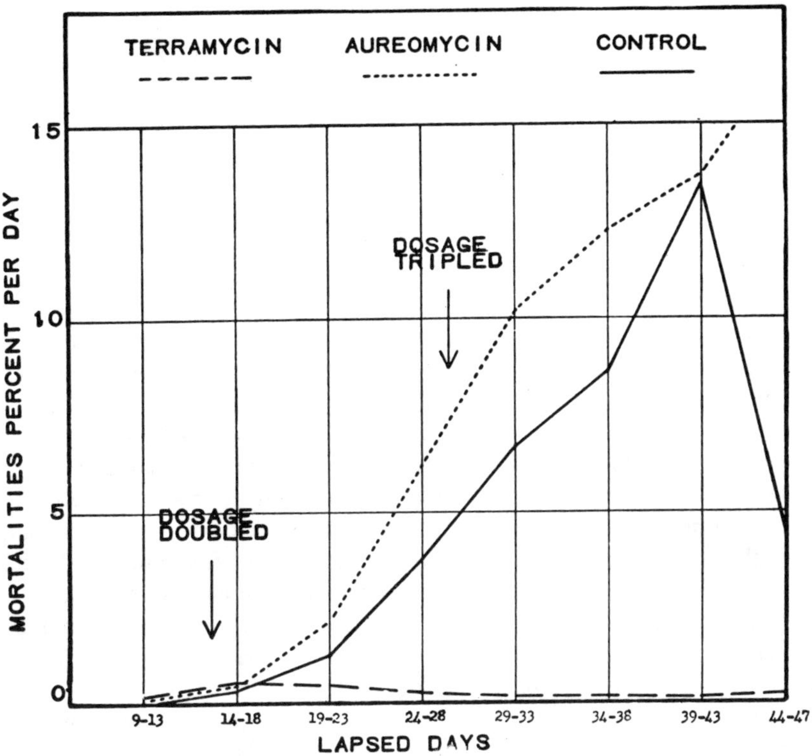


Figure 10. Ulcer disease. Mortalities of fingerling brook trout treated with antibiotics. Starting dosage 25 milligrams per kilogram of fish per day. (Snieszko, Griffin and Friddle, 1952)

milligrams per kilogram of body weight per day. The substitution of chloramphenicol for oxytetracycline would lessen the chances of appearance of oxytetracycline resistant forms of *H. piscium*.

In summary, control of ulcer disease may be achieved by treating infected fish with oxytetracycline at the rate of 75 milligrams per kilogram of body weight per day for ten to fifteen days or until the epizootic is brought under control. If necessary chloramphenicol at the same dosage rate may be given the last four or five days of the treatment period.

# Myxobacterioses

## Introduction

Myxobacterioses are probably the most common and widely occurring diseases of freshwater fishes. Outbreaks were also observed in river estuaries and bays containing salt water and marine fishes (Anderson and Conroy, 1969b). Lesions containing myxobacteria are almost without exception present in Pacific salmonids returning to spawn in freshwater. In many salmon and trout hatcheries regular preventive treatments are needed to control myxobacterial diseases. In warmwater ponds, rivers, or reservoirs, explosive fish epizootics caused by myxobacteria are often observed during summer when the water is low and the temperature high. Fish pathogenic myxobacteria are long, thin rods (2-10μ × 0.5–0.75μ). Taxonomically they belong to the family Cytophagaceae, genus *Cytophaga* and family Myxococcaceae, genus *Chondrococcus* (*Bergey's Manual* 7th edition Breed, *et al.*, 1957). The taxonomic position of myxobacteria is based in part on their ability to form fruiting bodies and microcysts. This is not satisfactory because formation of the resting stages of bacteria is influenced by many factors (Borg, 1960; Dworkin, 1966). There are at least three fish diseases attributed to myxobacteria. Perhaps the best known of these is columnaris disease, which is caused by a fruiting myxobacterium classified as *Chondrococcus columnaris*. The disease is most prevalent if water temperature is above the optimum temperature for fishes and affects both warm- and coldwater species of fishes. According to Garnjobst (1945) columnaris disease is also caused by *Cytophaga columnaris*. Coldwater, or peduncle disease, is caused by a non-fruiting myxobacterium *Cytophaga psychrophila*. The condition is most prevalent at temperatures below the optimum for *C. columnaris* and affects only salmonids. Myxobacteria either cause or are closely associated with a disease of juvenile salmonids termed bacterial gill disease. Whether one or more species of myxobacteria is involved in this disease is not known at the present. Various myxobacteria also occur in open lesions around fins or in the body musculature and it is almost impossible to decide if they are the primary etiologic agents or secondary invaders.

Perhaps one reason why relatively little work has been done with pathogenic myxobacteria has been their apparent lack of pathogenicity for man.

Recently, however, an anaerobic myxobacterium was isolated from the human oral cavity. Its pathogenicity was tested on warmblooded laboratory animals. Bacteria reproduced in lacerated tissues causing inflammation and ulceration (Graf, 1963a, 1963b). An excellent review of the biology of the myxobacteria (Dworkin, 1966) and a short review of the fish pathogenic myxobacteria (Anderson and Conroy, 1969b) have been published.

## Columnaris Disease

### INTRODUCTION

Columnaris disease was the first described disease of any animal caused by a pathogen belonging to the myxobacteria group (Davis, 1922). Myxobacteria were known since 1897 (Thaxter) but were known as saprophytes in soils rich in organic matter. Since its first description (Davis, 1922), columnaris disease has been observed in most species of freshwater and anadromous fishes and contributes to mortalities of salmon returning to freshwater for spawning. Marine fishes are also affected by myxobacterial diseases probably of the columnaris type.

As will be discussed in more detail, the causative agent of columnaris disease is of particular interest because of the great variability in virulence among strains and the possibility of its existing in both fruiting and non-fruiting forms.

### DEFINITION

Columnaris disease is a common disease of freshwater and possibly of marine fishes and is caused by myxobacteria described as *Chondrococcus columnaris* and *Cytophaga columnaris*. Another common fish disease described as coldwater, low temperature, or peduncle disease is, according to the present state of knowledge, caused by a different form of myxobacterium (*Cytophaga psychrophila*).

### HISTORICAL

The first description of columnaris disease was by Davis (1922) at the Fairport, Iowa, Fisheries Research Station;he observed outbreaks of a new disease among many species of warmwater fishes in aquaria, ponds, and under wild conditions. He described the symptoms, pathology, and histopathology of the disease and observed, but did not isolate, the pathogen. Davis named the pathogen *Bacillus columnaris* because the organisms in material removed from the lesion and observed microscopically in a wet mount were seen arranging themselves into dome shaped columns (Fig. 11).

A similar disease of salmonids was described by Ordal and Rucker (1944) and Fish and Rucker (1945) who recognized the etiologic agent as a myxobacterium, because of the flexibility of cells, production of globular microcysts, and very simple, or rudimentary, fruiting bodies. They called their isolate *Chondrococcus columnaris*. At about the same time, Garnjobst (1945) in Davis' laboratory at Leetown, West Virginia Fisheries Station, studied

Davis' original isolate and classified it as *Cytophaga columnaris* because she did not observe formation of microcysts. However a photograph in her paper suggests that forms which she considered as degenerative are strikingly similar to typical myxobacterial microcysts (Fig. 12).

Probably the most detailed description of myxobacterial fish diseases is that by Borg which was first written as an unpublished Ph.D. thesis in 1948, and in 1960 was published in microcard form. This report, as well as the reports by Ordal and Rucker (1944) and Garnjobst (1945), are probably the most complete on fish pathogenic myxobacteria.

### SYMPTOMS AND PATHOLOGY

The first external sign of columnaris disease is the appearance of grayish-white spots on the body of the fish, often on the head, lips, or fins. Superficially these spots are very similar to those caused by *Saprolegnia*. Sometimes tufts or flakes of epithelium and bacteria are loosely attached to the

Figure 11. *Chondrococcus columnaris* "column formation" on fish tissue. ×680. (Davis, 1946).

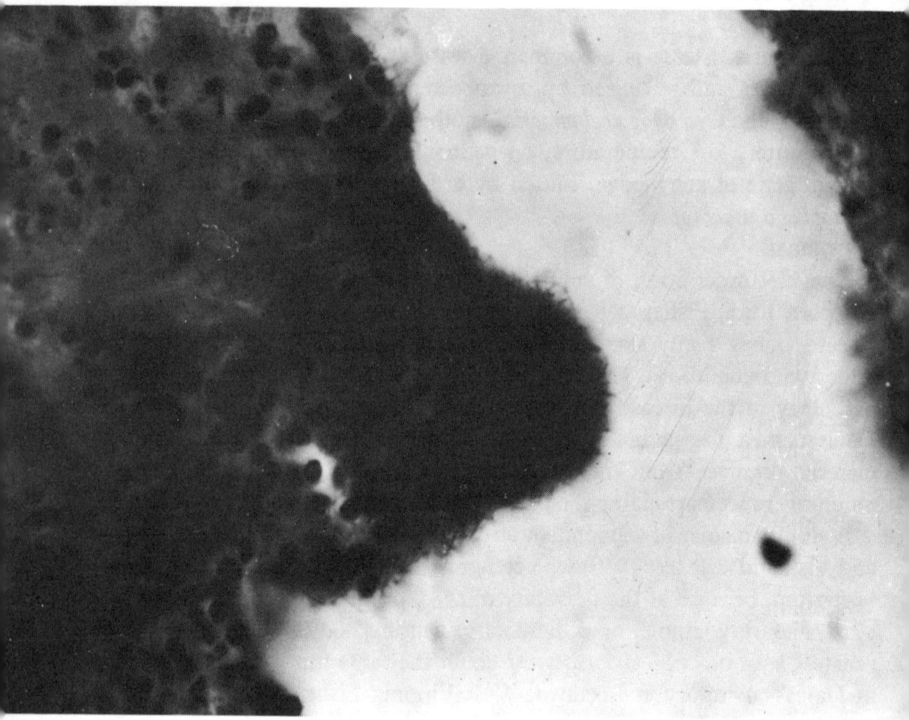

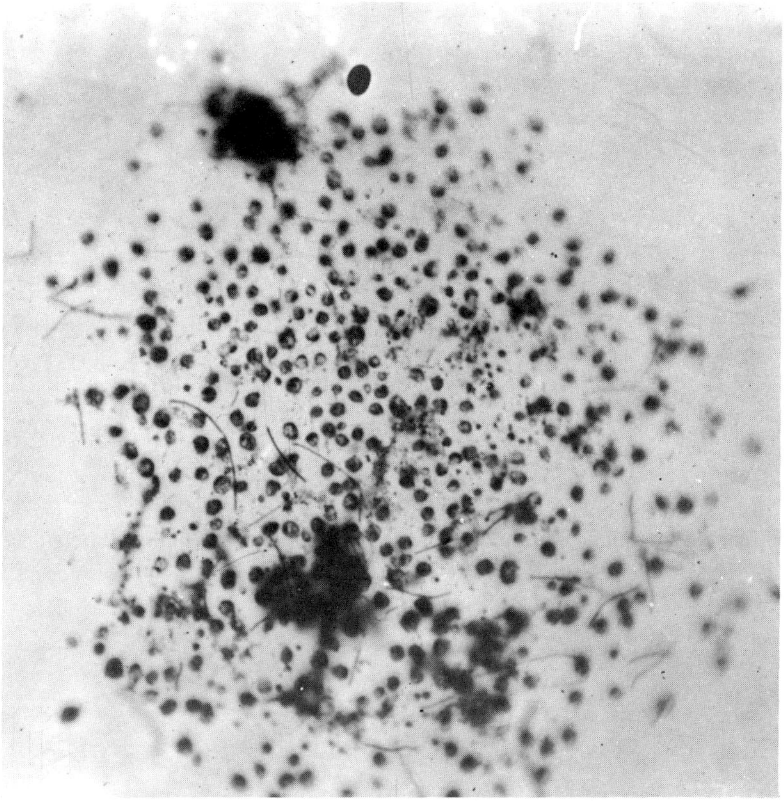

Figure 12. Stained smear of *Chondrococcus columnaris* showing vegetative cells and what appear to be microcysts ×680. (Garnjobst, 1945).

mouths of fishes and appear like tiny wads of cotton. For this reason aquarists often call columnaris disease "cotton wool disease" or "mouth fungus." Since it is not a fungus disease, this name should be discarded (van Duijn, 1967).

The external lesions are different on fishes without scales from those with scales. In scaleless fishes, such as bullheads or catfishes, the initial lesions are small and circular with grayish-blue centers and red margins surrounded by a ring of inflamed skin. When the disease progresses, irregular areas of skin are necrotic, grayish in appearance with small flakes of tissue dangling in water (Fig. 13). When the fish is removed from water these flakes collapse, adhere to the body, and are hard to see.

In scaled fishes, the initial visible lesion appears on the outer margins of fins as grayish-white discoloration consisting of proliferating epithelium

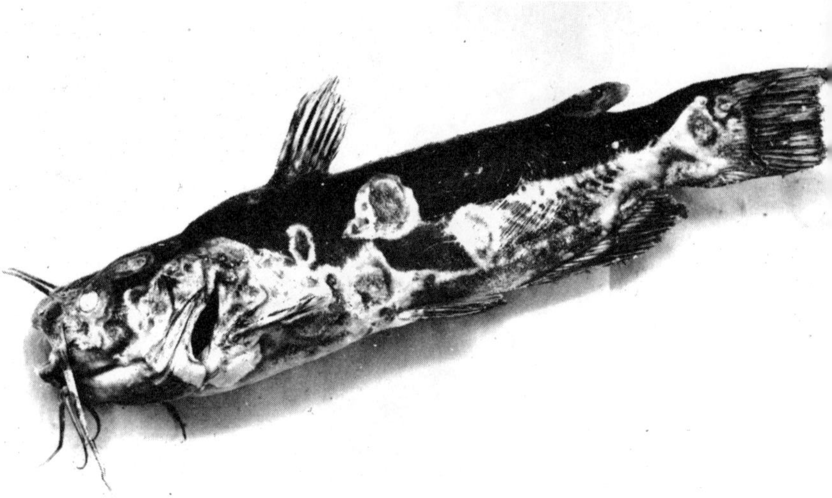

Figure 13. Advanced columnaris disease lesions on black bullhead (*Ictalurus melas*). (Davis, 1922)

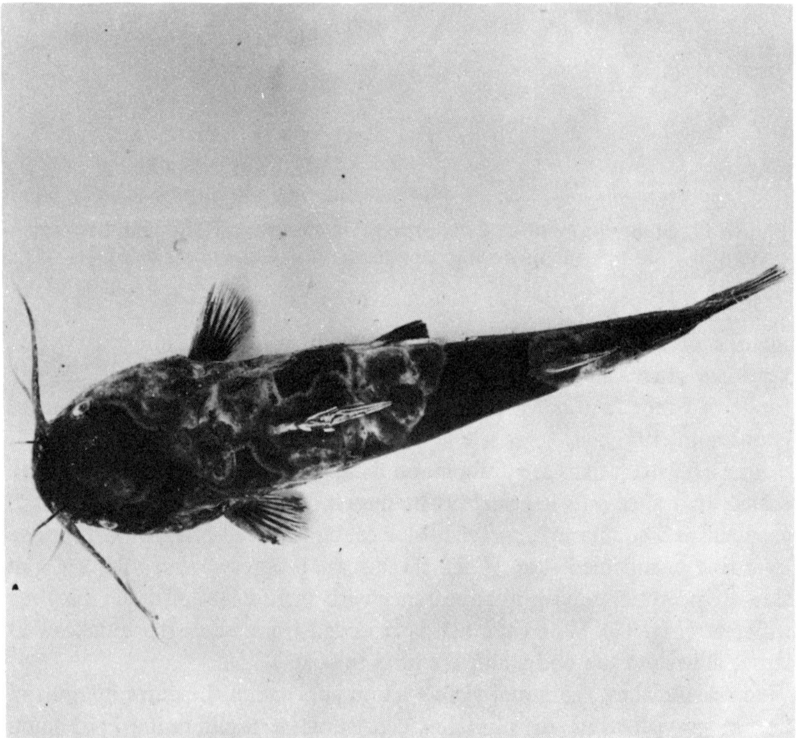

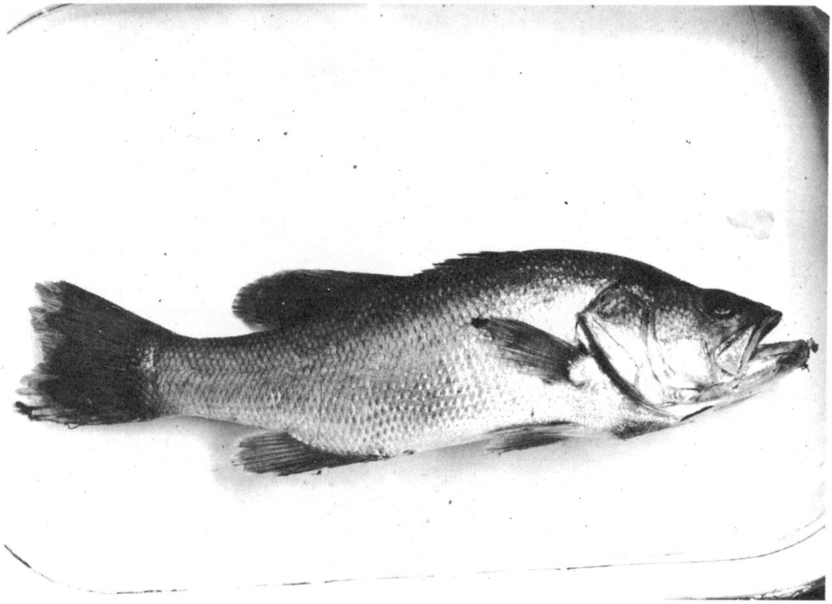

Figure 14. White bass (*Roccus chrysops*) and largemouth bass (*Micropterus salmoides*) showing fins with columnaris lesions. (Davis, 1922)

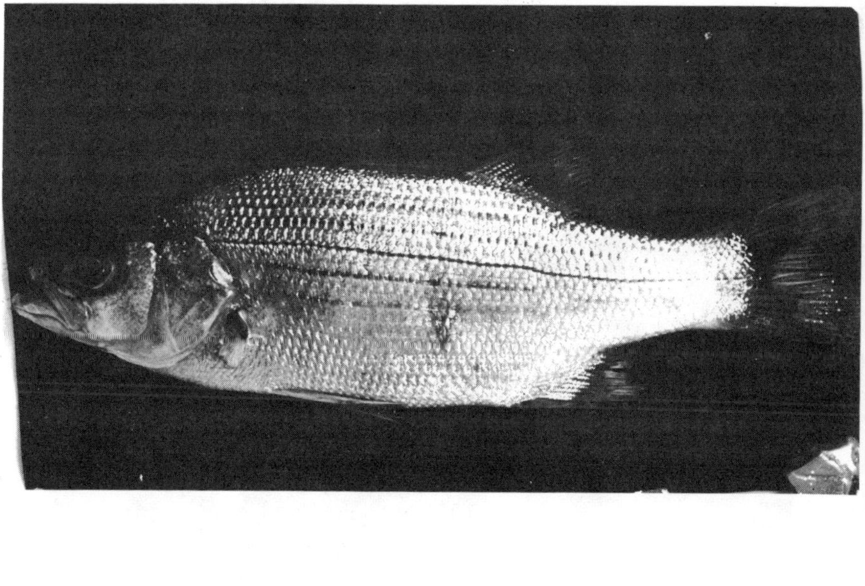

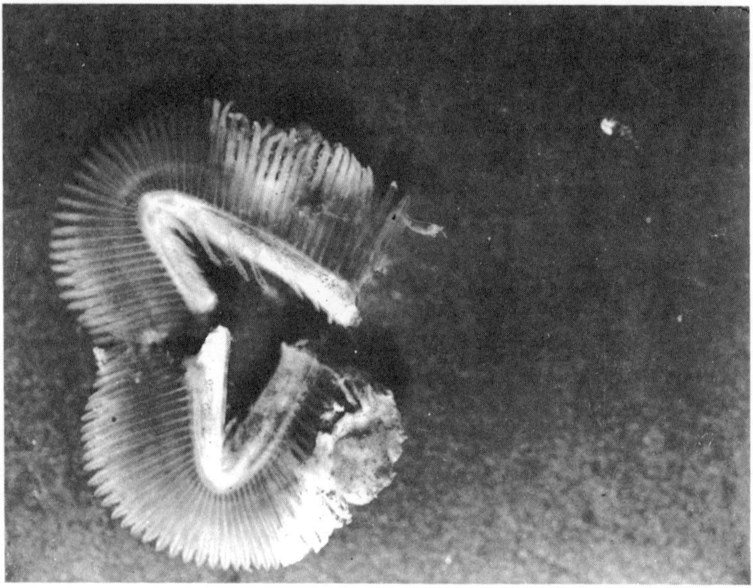

Whole gill arches.

Figure 15. Localized necrotic lesion of gill tissue caused by *Chondrococcus columnaris*.

Hematoxylin and eosin stained section of gill filaments. ×70.

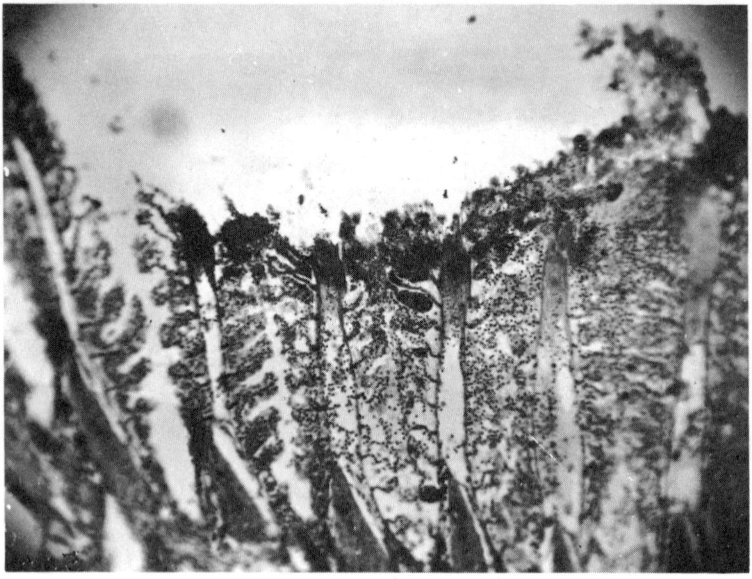

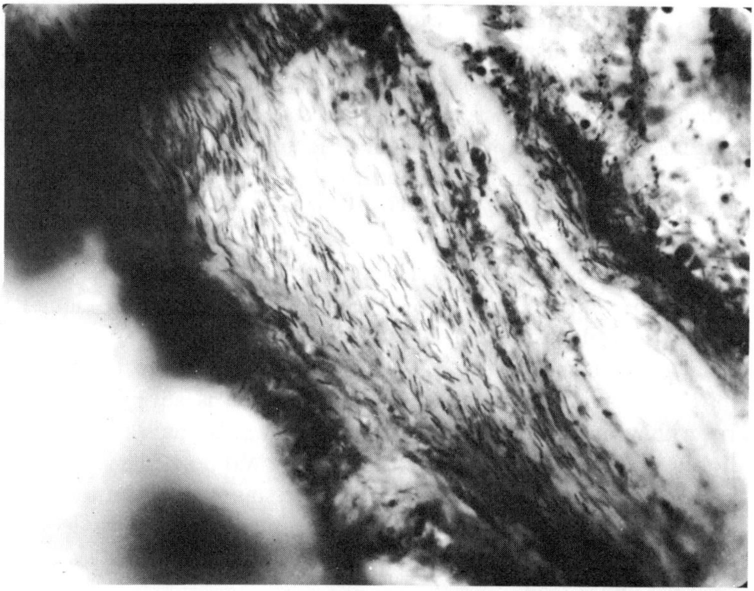

Figure 16. Stained smear of tissue infected with *Chondrococcus columnaris* showing an almost continuous sheet of myxobacteria. ×680.

and bacterial cells (Fig. 14). Gradually the lesions spread to the body of the fish and it appears to be covered with patches of mucus. A localized lesion often develops on the gills. Soft gill tissue becomes eroded, showing necrotic gaps (Fig. 15).

In smears and sections prepared from the affected tissues, typical myxobacteria are present. On the surface of the lesion, there is an almost continuous film of myxobacteria (Fig. 16). With skin lesions, bacteria are less numerous in the underlying tissues comprising the corium. Davis (1922) did not report on the presence of myxobacteria in internal organs of diseased fishes. In an outbreak of columnaris disease in blueback salmon (*O. nerka*) fingerlings at Leavenworth, Washington, Ordal and Rucker (1944) found the causative agent of the disease (*Chondrococcus columnaris*) also in internal organs. They observed systemic infections in several species of salmonid and other fishes taken from the Columbia River. Organisms could be isolated in pure culture from internal organs. No mention was made by Ordal and Rucker (1944) of any visible pathology of the invaded organs.

According to Fish and Rucker (1945), a hemorrhagic area usually appears at the anterior confluence of the branchiostegal rays. The gill tissue reacts at first to the infection with epithelial hyperplasia which is followed by sloughing and necrosis of the lamellae and finally of the central cartilaginous structures of the filaments. It should be noted that the difference between the myxobacterial gill disease and gill lesions caused by columnaris disease is that in gill disease the pathology consists of proliferation of epithelium resulting in a variable degree of gill fusion, while in columnaris disease it results in gill necrosis and erosion (Fig. 15). Fish and Rucker (1945) consistently isolated *C. columnaris* from internal organs but gross foci of infection were not observed.

In a recent report, Wood (1968) indicated that *C. columnaris* enters skin through abrasions but even undamaged gills can be infected. Among Pacific salmonids, while in freshwater, the skin and gill lesions are very characteristic. Skin lesions are often yellow because of large masses of bacteria which contain yellow pigment. Sometimes there is advanced necrosis of jaws with remnants of eroded jaws hanging down. Bacteria appear systemically after extensive skin or gill necrosis. There was no evidence of any gross lesions in internal organs. In rapidly progressing cases when the temperature of water approaches 20°C, there are no external gross lesions but numerous bacteria are present systemically. The pathogenesis in such cases is not yet understood.

ETIOLOGY

There is no doubt columnaris disease is caused by a myxobacterium, but taxonomy, classification, and identification of myxobacteria possibly causing columnaris disease, as well as a precise definition of the disease itself, are still being disputed. In this text only *Chondrococcus columnaris* and *Cytophaga columnaris* are considered as etiologic agents of columnaris disease. *Cytophaga psychrophila* is considered on a tentative basis.

Most fishery workers agree that the causative agent of columnaris disease is *Chondrococcus columnaris* as described by Ordal and Rucker (1944). However, the possibility of the existence of another form of *C. columnaris*, or even of another species belonging to a different genus (*Cytophaga columnaris*) as described by Garnjobst (1945) cannot be ruled out. The fact that Ordal and Rucker (1944) found that their cultures produced microcysts and fruiting bodies led them to place the myxobacterium in the genus *Chondrococcus*, while the apparent failure of Garnjobst to find the fruiting structures led her to classify her isolates in the genus *Cytophaga*. The different observations concerning microcysts and fruiting bodies appear to be the only major difference between the Ordal and Rucker cultures and those of Garnjobst, but illustrations in her paper indicate that microcysts were formed but not recognized as such. Borg (1948, 1960) suggested two possibilities to explain the different results: (1) Garnjobst was using cultures which, because of repeated subcultivation, had lost their ability to form microcysts and fruiting bodies; (2) there actually exist fruiting and non-fruiting forms of the same bacterium. Since the question of taxonomy is not at present resolvable, and because most columnaris outbreaks are caused by the form producing microcysts, we accept that the prime etiological agent of columnaris disease is *Chondrococcus columnaris*. However, one should be aware that non-fruiting strains could be encountered in columnaris disease.

### DIAGNOSIS

Diagnosis of a myxobacterial infection can be made on the basis of observing long, thin gram-negative rods in lesions or in internal organs. In wet mounts made with material removed from an open lesion, one can usually see the gradual gliding and oscillating motions of myxobacteria which in a few minutes may form a typical column (Fig. 11). When isolated and cultivated these bacteria form yellow pigmented, gliding colonies on Ordal's agar. Positive diagnosis of columnaris disease is based on identification of *C. columnaris* which may be accomplished by cultural and serological procedures to be discussed in a separate chapter.

### TRANSMISSION, EPIZOOTIOLOGY AND PATHOGENESIS

According to Davis (1922) transmission of the disease is facilitated by crowding, handling, and water temperatures above 25°C (77°F). If fish with open lesions are handled first and healthy fish soon afterwards, infection is transmitted by hands or tools. Any handling of pondfishes at 25°C or higher may result in outbreaks of columnaris. Breaking off scales opens portals of infection. When the disease is transferred by handling, the incubation period is one to two days. When disease subsides, repeated handling may result in another outbreak. The caudal peduncle in salmonids and warmwater fishes is particularly vulnerable to infection by handling. Fijan (1968) found that *C. columnaris* can survive for at least eight days in natural and reconstituted water of different hardness and pH, therefore transmission via the water route may add to the disease incidence in areas of sparcely populated streams.

There are numerous reports on the difference of virulence among different strains of *C. columnaris*. Davis observed that a larger percentage of positive results was obtained in infection experiments when material was taken from a fish of the same species. Pacha and Ordal (1963) and Wood (1968) reported on a considerable difference in the virulence of *C. columnaris* isolated from salmonids in the Columbia River and its tributaries. Presumably the differences in virulence are associated with toxins because infections caused by less virulent bacteria resulted in extensive tissue damage, gills in particular. Virulent strains caused losses without the presence of gross tissue damage. In Pacific salmonids very virulent strains caused infection and disease at 15°C (60°F) while less virulent strains caused outbreaks when the temperature reached 20°C (68°F) or above (J. Wood, 1968).

The age of the fishes is an important factor in susceptibility. Young fishes, during the first months of their lives, are much more susceptible and adults are more resistant or nearly immune (as observed in carp by Davis, 1922). Davis also believed that adult fishes resistant to infection were most likely to be the carriers of this pathogen.

The progress of columnaris disease is variable. In warmwater fishes in ponds, rivers, or lakes, columnaris disease is often explosive during the time of the year when the temperature of water reaches the maximum level for the season. In such cases there are extensive necrotic areas of the dermis but without any gross internal pathology. It may be assumed that in such cases the death of the fishes is caused by loss of electrolytes and proteins through the open lesions as is the case of salmon with coldwater disease. In systemic myxobacteriosis, death probably occurs as a result of bacterial toxins or toxins liberated by the body of the host under the highly proteolytic action of myxobacteria.

In cases wherein large areas of gills are necrotic or completely destroyed, death is probably caused by asphyxiation, partial loss of excretory function, and loss of plasma electrolytes and proteins through the open gill lesions.

### HOST AND GEOGRAPHIC RANGE

Columnaris disease is one of the most ubiquitous fish diseases known as affecting warmwater and coldwater species, scaled and scaleless species (Davis, 1953), as well as aquarium fishes (van Duijn, 1967; Axelrod, 1962) (Table 10). Unlike the other myxobacterial diseases which apparently are primarily limited to propagated fishes, columnaris disease occurs in fishes in both the hatchery and natural habitat (Rucker, Earp and Ordal, 1954; Bottomley and Holland, 1966). The disease is particularly serious to Pacific

TABLE 10. Species of fishes from which columnaris disease has been described.

(Anderson and Conroy, 1969b) Modified.

| Fish species | | Author(s) |
|---|---|---|
| *Family*: Clupeidae | | |
| Gizzard shad | *(Dorosoma cepedianum)* | Isom (1960) |
| *Family*: Salmonidae | | |
| Sockeye salmon | *(Oncorhynchus nerka)* | Fish and Rucker (1945) |
| Chinook salmon | *(O. tschawytscha)* | Johnson and Brice (1953) |
| Coho salmon | *(O. kisutch)* | ,, ,, ,, ,, |
| Pink salmon | *(O. gorbuscha)* | Fish and Rucker (1945) |
| Rainbow trout / Steelhead trout | *(Salmo gairdneri)* | Rucker *et al.* (1954) |
| Cutthroat trout | *(S. clarki)* | Johnson and Brice (1953) |
| Brook trout | *(Salvelinus fontinalis)* | Davis (1946) |
| Mountain whitefish | *(Prosopium williamsoni)* | Rucker *et al.* (1954) |

| Fish species | | Author(s) |
|---|---|---|
| *Family*: Catostomidae | | |
| Smallmouth buffalo | *(Ictiobus bubalus)* | Davis (1922) |
| Bigmouth buffalo | *(I. cyprinellus)* | ,, ,, |
| Northern hog sucker | *(Hypentelium nigricans)* | Lennon and Parker (1960) |
| Flathead catfish | *(Pylodictis olivaris)* | ,, ,, |
| *Family*: Cyprinidae | | |
| Carp | *(Cyprinus carpio)* | Isom (1960) |
| Roach | *(Rutilus rutilus)* | Ajmal and Hobbs (1967) |
| Northern sqauwfish | *(Ptychocheilus oregonensis)* | Rucker *et al.* (1953) |
| Stoneroller | *(Campostoma anomalum)* | Lennon and Parker (1960) |
| Bluntnose minnow | *(Pimephales notatus)* | Davis (1922) |
| *Family*: Ictaluridae | | |
| Blue catfish | *(Ictalurus furcatus)* | Isom (1960) |
| Channel catfish | *(I. punctatus)* | Davis (1922) |
| Black bullhead | *(I. melas)* | ,, ,, |
| Brown bullhead | *(I. nebulosus)* | Garnjobst (1945) |
| Flat bullhead | *(Ictalurus platycephalus)* | Nigrelli (1943) |
| *Family*: Cyprinodontidae | | |
| Mummichog | *(Fundulus heteroclitus)* | Nigrelli and Hutner (1945) |
| *Family*: Serranidae | | |
| White bass | *(Roccus chrysops)* | Davis (1922) |
| *Family*: Centrarchidae | | |
| Smallmouth bass | *(Micropterus dolomieui)* | Isom (1960) |
| Largemouth bass | *(M. salmoides)* | ,, ,, |
| Bluegill | *(Lepomis macrochirus)* | ,, ,, |
| Orangespotted sunfish | *(L. humilis)* | Davis (1922) |
| Sunfish | *(L. incisor)* | ,, ,, |
| Warmouth | *(Chaenobryttus gulosus)* | ,, ,, |
| White crappie | *(Pomoxis annularis)* | ,, ,, |
| Crappie | *(P. sparoides)* | ,, ,, |
| *Family*: Percidae | | |
| Perch | *(Perca fluviatilis)* | Ajmal and Hobbs (1967) |
| Yellow perch | *(P. flavescens)* | Davis (1922) |
| *Family*: Cobitidae | | |
| Japanese weather fish | *(Misgurnus anguilli-caudatus)* | Wakabayashi and Egusa (1967) |

salmon fingerlings migrating to the sea and to returning salmon (Colgrove and Wood, 1966). It is a very serious disease of propagated scaleless fishes such as buffalofishes (*Ictiobus bubalus* and *Megastomatobus cyprinella*) (Davis, 1953) and aquarium fishes such as black mollies (Axelrod, 1962).

Colgrove and Wood (1966) state that "columnaris disease occurs only in fresh water," and this is supported by the lack of reports of columnaris disease in marine and estuarine fishes. However myxobacterial infections, which are columnaris-like in their external pathology, have occurred occasionally in marine and estuarine fishes. For example, Borg (1948, 1960) isolated a myxobacterium from caudal lesions of pink salmon (*Onchorynchus gorbuscha*) in saltwater. He found the isolate resembled *C. columnaris* in swarming activity but the individual cells were longer than those of *C. columnaris*. A myxobacterium was also implicated in an epizootic of white perch (*Roccus americanus*) in the brackish water of Chesapeake Bay. Again the myxobacterium resembled *C. columnaris* but failed to react with *C. columnaris* antiserum.

Observations made in southern states (Snow and Camper, pers. comm.) have shown that frog tadpoles were susceptible to columnaris disease. The possible role of frogs as carriers of fish pathogenic myxobacteria is an open question.

Columnaris disease has been most often reported in freshwater fishes of North America, and more recently in Japan (Wakabayashi and Egusa, 1967). Borg (1948, 1960) observed symptoms of columnaris disease in pink salmon reared in saltwater fish hatcheries. Myxobacteria were abundant in lesions but proved very fastidious. Myxobacterial diseases of marine fishes are not listed in the recent review on diseases of marine fishes (Sindermann, 1966, 1970). A condition of rainbow trout maintained in salt water, "eroded mouth," is discussed by Anderson and Conroy (1969b). The disease was external and destroyed the epidermis and much of the dermis, exposing cartilaginous tissue. Vast numbers of myxobacteria could be seen in the dermis. The organism grew poorly on initial isolation, but grew better after several subcultures. Dipping affected fish in 1:200 copper sulfate (prepared with fresh water) successfully cured the disease.

An outbreak of a disease affecting white perch in Chesapeake Bay occurred during the summer of 1965, causing considerable mortality. Fish displayed dermal lesions typical for columnaris disease and myxobacteria were present in the necrotic areas. The disease was tentatively diagnosed as columnaris disease but a precise taxonomic identification of the myxobacterium was not established.

### CONTROL MEASURES

Columnaris disease is common among freshwater and marine fishes, is capable of causing great losses, and is therefore of considerable economic importance. Because of this, various methods of prevention and treatment were investigated.

#### *Treatment*

As early as 1918, Davis (1922) tested the efficacy of potassium permanganate and copper sulfate. Because of their low cost, these chemicals could be used economically for treatment of large numbers of fishes in great volumes of water. Unfortunately both chemicals are toxic to most fish species and the margin of safety is narrow. Buffalofishes, which are very susceptible to columnaris disease, are also very sensitive to these chemicals. The highest concentration of potassium permanganate safe for buffalofishes and still effective for treatment was 1:50,000 for ten to fifteen minutes. Black bass and bluegills could be treated safely with a solution of 1:20,000 for the same length of time.

Copper sulfate was recommended by Davis (1922) in concentration of 1:30,000 for twenty minutes. Immediately after treatment, fishes should be placed in flowing water. According to Davis, "It should be distinctly borne in mind that the treatment to be effective must be given within a few hours after the fish have been handled and before any signs of infection appear. If the fish are to be confined in aquaria, two or three successive treatments at 12 to 24 hour intervals are advisable. When this treatment is properly used it is believed it will effectually prevent any serious outbreak of the disease. It must be repeated, however, every time the fish are handled or subjected to injury in any way."

Treatment of columnaris disease in aquarium fishes may be accomplished with various drugs or chemicals. Van Duijn (1967) recommends the following treatments:

1. Brilliant green water solution containing 65 p.p.m. Dipping for forty-five seconds. Treatment is effective but dangerous to fishes.
2. Hydrogen peroxide. A solution is prepared containing 20 ml of commercial 3% solution of peroxide for 1 liter of water. Fishes are introduced to this solution for ten to fifteen minutes. Repeated daily treatments are recommended.
3. Chloramphenicol (chloromycetin) and chlortetracycline (Aureomycin) added to aquarium water at a concentration of 10–20 p.p.m. are usually effective. For stubborn cases, concentration of 100 p.p.m. is recommended. Both antibiotics may be toxic to aquarium plants.

According to J. Wood (1968), hatchery-raised Pacific salmon given prolonged treatment, one hour, with pyridylmercuric acetate technical (P.M.A.) at a concentration of 1–2 p.p.m. gave satisfactory results in case of external infections. Recently PMA has been replaced by Diquat (2–4 p.p.m. of Diquat cation) which has to be used for four consecutive days.

The most effective chemotherapeutic drug for systemic infection is oxytetracycline given orally with food at a rate of 8–10 grams per 100 kg fish per day (4 g/100 lb/day) for ten days. Combined external and systemic treatments give longer lasting results. Quarternary ammonia compounds and sulfonamides have very small beneficial effect.

Lowering of temperature to below 15°C (60°F) is very effective in prevention and even cure of columnaris disease in Pacific salmonids.

## Peduncle and Coldwater Disease

### DEFINITION

It seems that coldwater (or low temperature) disease and peduncle disease of salmonids are two different names of the same disease. Both forms of this disease affect salmonids when the water temperature is below 10°C. Both forms are characterized by typical external lesions and terminate as systemic infections with similar pathology. A serological comparison of coldwater disease and peduncle disease isolates at the Eastern Fish Disease Laboratory showed they have common agglutinins and precipitins. The main difference is that coldwater disease causes large mortalities in juvenile Pacific salmon whereas peduncle disease is a mild disease of fingerling or yearling trout on the east coast of the United States. The two diseases will be considered as one, and the term peduncle disease will be used in this text. For a complete description of the disease in coho salmon, the reader is referred to Wood (1968).

### HISTORICAL

The first description of peduncle disease was made by Davis (1946) who observed the condition in fingerling rainbow trout at the Leetown (West Virginia) National Hatchery. It ended invariably in death of trout. The diseased tissue contained long thin (3–5μ) bacteria. A low temperature disease of salmonids (coldwater disease) was described by Borg (1948, 1960) who observed it in silver salmon fingerling in the state of Washington. At times this disease destroyed up to one-third of the fingerling salmon but it is not very common in trout.

### SYMPTOMS AND PATHOLOGY

In trout the first area affected is usually the adipose fin which becomes white along the outer edge. The discoloration extends gradually toward the base until the entire fin is discolored. Eventually the entire caudal peduncle becomes a dirty-white, the adipose fin is destroyed, and the integument on the dorsal side of the peduncle disintegrates, exposing the muscle. Necrosis of muscle tissue continues and the vertebral column may be exposed before the fish dies (Davis, 1946) (Fig. 17). With salmon, lesions may begin on the adopose fin, on the isthmus, or on the back, anterior to the dorsal fin. In some cases no apparent surface lesions occur and salmon show a darkening before death (Borg, 1948, 1960). In coho salmon (Wood and Yasutake, 1956a) the most consistently infected areas were the head, particularly the mouth, and the kidney. In various individuals massive concentrations of myxobacteria occurred in the heart, peritoneum, and spleen. In the gills myxobacteria were found in small capillaries in the respiratory lamellae, and in the kidney the organism had an affinity for renal glomeruli, with glomerular capillaries often containing solid masses of myxobacteria. Tubules leading from the affected glomeruli were in various stages of necrosis and

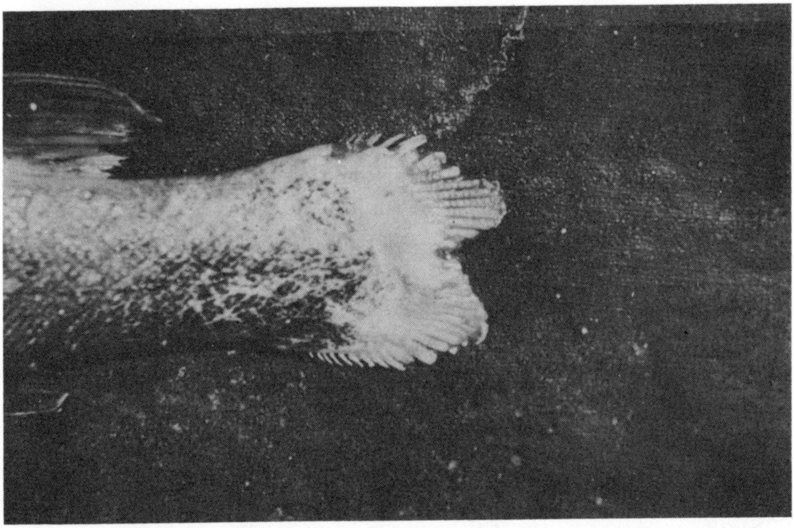

Figure 17. Advanced coldwater disease in brook trout (*Salvelinus fontinalis*) yearling. (This figure, reproduced in color, appears after Index.)

degeneration. Individual muscle fibers of the heart were attacked, causing slight inflammation and necrosis. In infected chinook salmon fingerlings, histological examination showed myxobacteria present only in the gills. This confirmed previous bacteriological findings in that coldwater disease was septicemic in coho salmon; but in fingerling chinook salmon, myxobacteria could be seen and isolated only from the gills (Rucker *et al.*, 1954).

ETIOLOGY

Peduncle disease is caused by a gram-negative, yellow pigmented rod with an average size of 3.5μ × 0.75μ. The characteristics of the several isolates were originally studied by Borg (1948, 1960) and more recently by Pacha (1968), and the organism is presently classified as *Cytophaga psychrophila* (Borg) because microcyst formation in this myxobacterium was not observed. Strains isolated from eastern and western United States have shown many common morphological and biochemical properties as well as serological similarities.

DIAGNOSIS

Tentative diagnosis of peduncle disease may be made on the basis of symptoms and the occurrence of a myxobacterial infection when water temperatures are very cold (10–12°C) (50–54°F). Since salmonids with peduncle disease and advanced tail rot may show similar gross pathology, definitive diagnosis of peduncle disease is based on isolation and identification of *C. psychrophila.*

TRANSMISSION AND PATHOGENESIS

Transmission of peduncle disease is probably fish to fish, from wild carrier fish in hatchery water supply (Wood, 1968). Transovarian transmission in coho salmon has been suspected but not proved.

Pacha (1968) postulated that the proteolytic nature of *C. psychrophila* plays a part in the mode of pathogenesis and this would be probable because of the tissue damage usually seen in the disease. However, once the bacteria have become systemic, endotoxins may also play a part in the pathogenesis.

HOST AND GEOGRAPHIC RANGE

Among cultured fishes, peduncle disease is limited to salmonids. Coho salmon fingerlings are most susceptible, but sockeye and chinook salmon may also become diseased. As previously mentioned, the disease is milder in trout and most cases of peduncle disease occur in eastern brook trout.

The reported range is the continental United States, particularly in the northeast and northwest.

CONTROL

*Prevention*

The most effective means of preventing coldwater disease in young salmon is to reduce the stocking density or to rear the young salmon in troughs inside (where water temperatures are warmer) until mid-April coupled with a prophylactic feeding of sulfamethazine at the rate of 4.4 grams per 100 kilograms of fish per day until the temperature goes above 10°C. Of course, strict sanitation procedures described in previous sections are important in controlling outbreaks. Rearing coho salmon fry in shallow troughs reduces the severity of outbreaks at hatcheries where the disease is prevalent (Wood, 1968).

*Treatment*

Treatment of coldwater disease in Pacific salmonids differs from treatment of other bacterial diseases in that it is really a combination of therapy and prophylaxis. This is continued until the water temperature is higher than 10°C. Sulfamethazine had been used in what was named a 22–4.4–22 treatment. When the coho salmon start to feed they are fed a meat-meal diet containing a therapeutic dose of 22 grams per 100 kilograms of fish per day for ten days after which they receive a prophylactic dose of 4.4 grams per 100 kilograms of fish per day until seven days before they begin to receive the Oregon moist pellets, when they again receive the 22 gram level. Medicated Oregon moist pellets containing the prophylactic level of sulfamethazine are fed until the water temperature reaches a mean of 10°C. Recently sulfisoxazole and an experimental sulfonamide (sulfaethoxypyridazine) were tested for their ability to control coldwater disease. The above two drugs, along with sulfamethazine, were also tested for controlling coldwater disease using the 22–4.4–22 treatment and a continuous 8.8 grams per 100 kilograms of fish per day treatment. A hatchery with a high incidence of coldwater disease was chosen for the trials and the following results were obtained. All three drugs controlled peduncle disease when used at the continuous 4 gram level or the older 22–4.4–22 treatment method. However, sulfisoxazole and sulfaethoxypyridazine were more effective than sulfamethazine when used at the continuous 8.8 gram level (Amend, Fryer and Pilcher, 1965). If sulfisaxazole is approved for such use by the Food and Drug Administration, the continuous 8.8 gram level treatment with this drug is the most effective presently known. If the disease is not too advanced increasing water temperature to between 12°–15°C may suffice to control the disease (Wood, 1968).

## Bacterial Gill Disease

### INTRODUCTION

There are several types of gill disease in fishes. Bacterial gill disease is attributed to a combination of unfavorable environmental conditions with infection of the gills by myxobacteria. Nutritional gill disease is caused by a deficiency of panthotenic acid. "Hemorrhagic" gill disease is characterized by the presence of sand-grain size aneurysms in the gill capillaries and may be caused by chemical pollution, pesticides, or blood parasites. *Branchiomycosis* is an infection of the gills of pondfish caused by fungi belonging to the genus *Branchiomyces*. Pathological gill changes may also be caused by various toxic agents and unfavorable environmental conditions.

### DEFINITION

Bacterial gill disease is believed to be principally a myxobacterial infection which is preceded and triggered by unfavorable environmental conditions. The infection results in proliferation of gill epithelium and in extreme cases fusion of gill filaments (Fig. 18). Nutritional gill disease is symptomatically similar to bacterial gill disease and both types may occur at the same time. In such cases, diagnosis and establishment of etiology are very difficult.

This section will be devoted chiefly to the description of bacterial gill disease, however some aspects of nutritional gill disease will be covered because of its similarity to bacterial gill disease. Hemorrhagic gill disease and gill rot will be discussed in their appropriate sections.

### HISTORICAL

Although earlier reports of gill pathology similar to that seen in bacterial gill disease exist, the first mention of the presence of bacteria, morphologically similar to myxobacteria, was given by Davis (1926). The outbreak affected fingerling brook and rainbow trouts at an experimental hatchery in Vermont. As the culture of salmonids became more intense bacterial gill disease has become a major cause of mortality in juvenile fishes. As far as can be determined, very few, if any, hatcheries propagating salmonids are free of outbreaks of bacterial gill disease.

SYMPTOMS AND PATHOLOGY

To the experienced hatcheryman, bacterial gill disease may be easily recognized on the basis of symptoms. Affected fishes suddenly stop feeding, appear sluggish, remain near the water surface, and often line up against the current near the water inlet. One of the most constant symptoms is the increased mucous secretions by the gills (Davis, 1953). Gills may also be swollen and congested which results in their appearing a deeper red than usual. In advanced cases gill lamellae are clubbed and filaments may be fused because of hyperplasia of gill epithelium (Fig. 18). Microscopic examination of infected gills reveals hyperplasia of the lamellae and the presence of myxobacteria, usually in groups (Figs. 19 and 20). Histological examination of infected gills showed a close relationship between the presence of myxobacteria and the increase in the number of epithelial cells. Structures similar to the plaque formation observed by Burrows (quoted in Rucker, *et al.*, 1952) were also observed by Wood and Yasutake (1957). However, Burrows thought the plaques were bacterial colonies whereas Wood and Yasutake (1957) described plaques as being composed of single

Figure 18. Advanced case of bacterial gill disease showing clubbing and fusing of lamellae and filaments. ×14. (Davis, 1946)

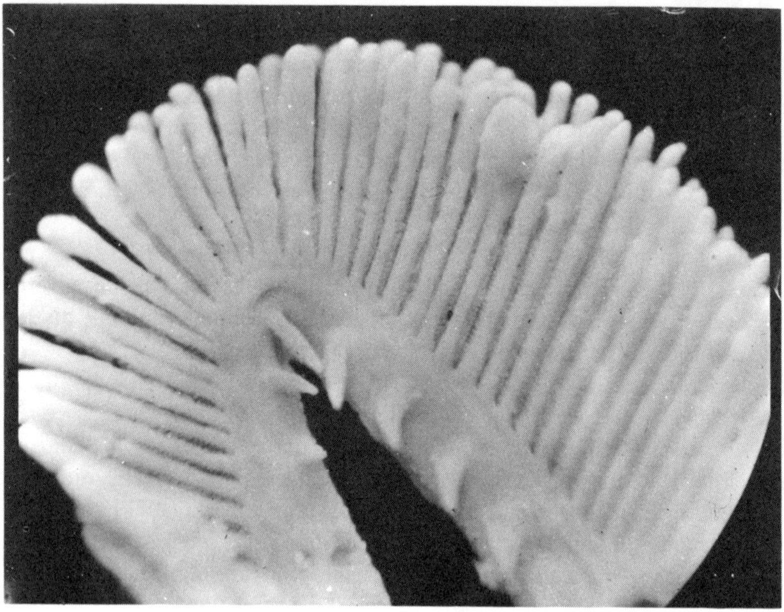

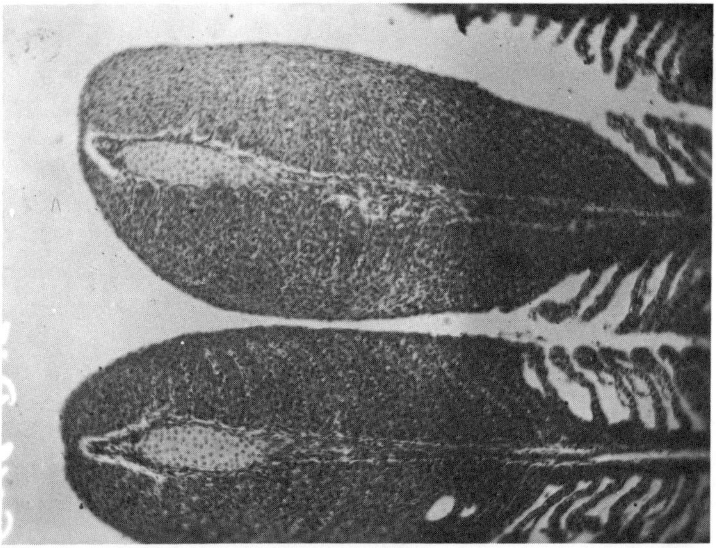

Approximately ×70.

Figure 19. Histological section of gill lamellae and filaments infected with gill myxobacteria. Note the fusion of lamellae at tips of the filaments. (Davis, 1946)

×25.

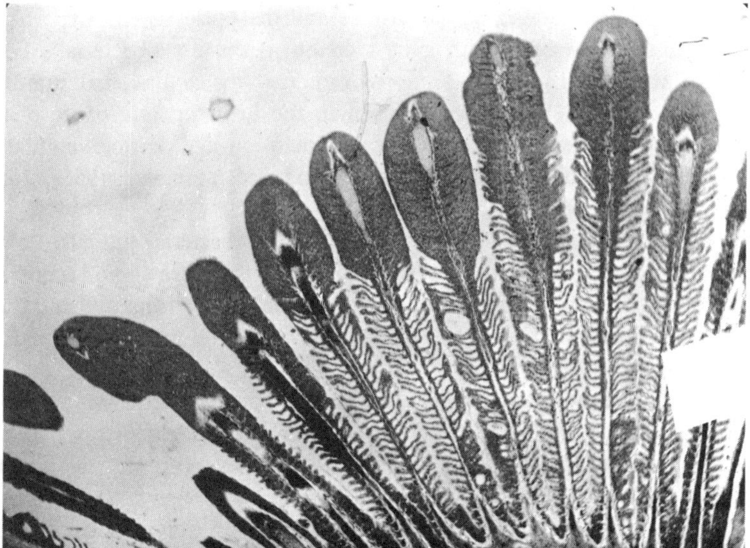

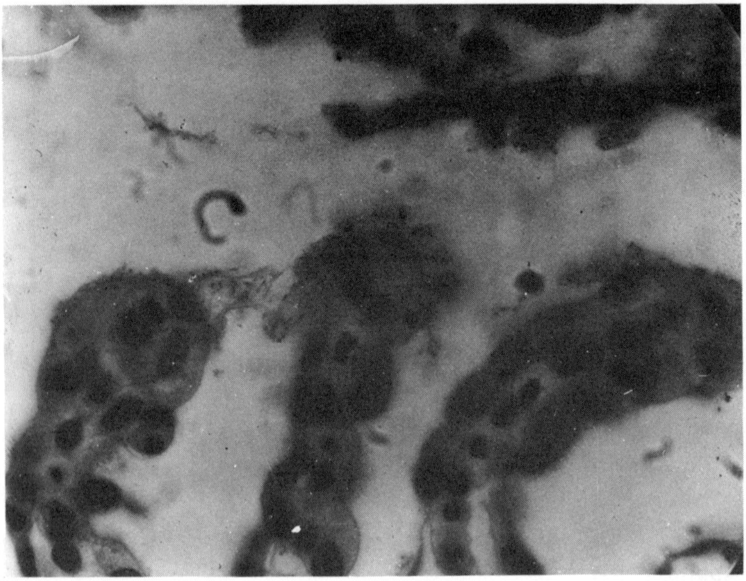

Figure 20. Masses of gill myxobacteria on the tips of swollen laemellae. ×680. (Davis, 1946)

globose cells projecting from the lamellae. The cells were filled with intensely basophilic granules. Both descriptions indicate that the plaques occur in the early stages of the disease and disappear as the hyperplasia develops, followed by an apparent increase in the myxobacteria. Myxobacteria were not observed in sections of internal organs, but small numbers of necrotic endothelial cells were seen in the hematopoetic tissue of the kidney. In the affected endothelial cells, inclusion-like particles similar to those described in coldwater disease (Wood and Yasutake, 1956a, 1957) were also seen.

It was mentioned earlier that nutritional and bacterial gill disease are very similar in gross symptoms. Histologically, there are some identifying characteristics which can be used to distinguish between the two and these are summarized in Table 11.

ETIOLOGY

There is good circumstantial evidence that myxobacteria (or a specific myxobacterium) are the etiologic agency of bacterial gill disease. Myxobacteria are seen in great numbers on gill surfaces in epizootics and they may be easily isolated from infected gills.

Since several different morphological types have been isolated, some investigators believe more than one species of myxobacteria are involved

TABLE 11. Histological differences of nutritional and bacterial gill disease (Wood and Yasutake, 1957).

| *Pathology* | *Bacterial gill disease* | *Nutritional gill disease* |
|---|---|---|
| Hyperplasia of lamellae | Yes | Yes |
| Hyperplasia at base of lamellae | No | Yes |
| Hyperplasia at tip of lamellae | Yes | No |
| Lesion start at distal end of filament | Sometimes | Yes |
| Affected lamellae shortened | No | Yes |
| Affected lamellae longer and bent | Yes | No |

in the disease process (Borg, 1948, 1960; Wood, 1968; Bullock, 1970). Even though several species may be involved, they all share the following general characteristics described by Borg (1948, 1960): long thin gram-negative rods (0.9–1.1μ × 3.0–8.5μ) which exhibit a swinging motion when attached to gill surfaces, and on semi-solid media form yellow colonies with spreading edges. Cultures have never been observed to form fruiting bodies or microcysts and, using the present classification, most isolates would be classified in the genus *Cytophaga*.

Although myxobacteria dominate in bacterial gill disease, large numbers of gram-negative eubacteria have been reported in gill lesions with the pathological changes in gill tissue attributed to these bacteria (Wood and Yasutake, 1957; Klinger, 1958). It is possible one or more species of eubacteria are involved along with myxobacteria in the etiology of gill disease.

Because bacterial gill disease may be effectively treated with external disinfectants, there is no doubt that bacteria are closely associated with the disease process. However, attempts in the early 1950's to infect healthy fish under good environmental conditions using either pure cultures of myxobacteria or infected gill tissues were unsuccessful (Rucker, Johnson and Kaydas, 1952). More recent attempts to transmit bacterial gill disease using pure culture or mixed culture of myxobacteria or infected gill tissue were also unsuccessful (Bullock, 1970). There apparently must be predisposing factors which trigger the infection and Burrows (1964) postulated that continuous exposure to metabolic ammonia was the precursor to bacterial gill disease. He also demonstrated that the amount of hyperplasia of lamellae in chinook salmon fingerling gills increased with an increase in the concentration of un-ionized ammonia. The effect of ammonia and low levels of dissolved oxygen on induction of bacterial gill disease has been experimentally examined. Fingerling rainbow trout were placed in four aquaria at the rate of 1 part of trout to 15 parts of water by volume. Water flow into two aquaria was adjusted to allow a complete change of water in approximately one hour. The slow exchange of water caused the

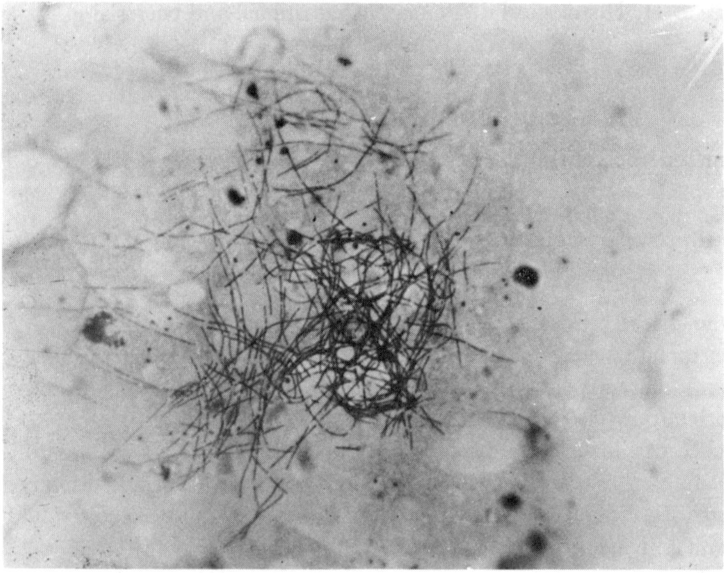

Figure 21. Stained smear of crushed, infected gill tissue showing masses of myxobacteria. ×680.

dissolved oxygen to drop to 4.0–4.5 p.p.m. and the ammonia level, measured as nesslerized ammonia, to rise to 1.0–1.5 p.p.m. The water exchange rate in the other two aquaria was rapid so that the oxygen level was 6.0–7.0 p.p.m. and no detectable ammonia was present. After ten to fourteen days under these conditions, trout in aquaria with low oxygen and high ammonia suffered an outbreak of bacterial gill disease, but no outbreaks occurred among trout in the other aquaria. The induction period could be shortened to three days if diseased fingerlings were added to aquaria with the slowly changing water. However, the experiment could not be repeated when the dissolved oxygen and ammonia levels were accurately controlled. This indicates that factors other than ammonia or oxygen may be involved and contribute to the complete chain of events triggering bacterial gill disease.

DIAGNOSIS

Tentative diagnosis of bacterial gill disease may be made on the basis of the behavioral symptoms described. Definitive diagnosis is based on the microscopic examination of gills for the presence of hyperplasia, swelling, clubbing and fusing of filaments and lamellae, and the presence of myxobacteria (Figs. 20 and 21). The myxobacteria may be observed in clumps near the tips of the filaments when gills are examined in wet mount under a magnification of 400–500 diameters. In severe cases the myxobacteria may form a continuous layer on the gill surface (Davis, 1953). Infected gill tissue may also be crushed and stained with a simple stain or by the Gram method. The masses as well as the individual cells may be more clearly seen in stained preparation (Fig. 21). Isolation of myxobacteria is not necessary for diagnosis because there are still no methods for conclusive identification of bacteria involved in gill disease.

### TRANSMISSION AND PATHOGENESIS

Myxobacteria are common bacteria in water and soil and probably continually surround the fish. Transmission of bacterial gill disease most likely occurs from water to fish in the beginning stages of an epizootic and then fish to fish transmission occurs as the disease spreads.

Hyperplasia of gill epithelium plus an increase in mucous production would seriously impair the free exchange of gases between the water and fish's blood, resulting in death of fish by asphyxiation.

### HOST AND GEOGRAPHIC RANGE

Bacterial gill disease is mainly a disease of hatchery raised salmonids but it also affects warmwater pondfishes (Davis, 1953). The selectivity for salmonids may be more apparent than real since environmental stress conditions probably trigger outbreaks and these conditions may occur more easily in tanks and raceways containing salmonids than in large ponds used for culture of warmwater species. Salmonids over 15 cm long do not regularly develop bacterial gill disease and the condition is more prevalent in juvenile fish.

Bacterial gill disease was for a time reported only from hatcheries in the United States. In 1958 an outbreak of bacterial gill disease was described in rainbow trout in Switzerland. However, in addition to gill disease, there was another septicemic infection involving a smaller gram-negative bacterium similar to *A. liquefaciens*. The smaller bacterium also occurred in large numbers on the gills (Klingler, 1958). Shortly thereafter a detailed report of bacterial gill disease in Portugal was given by Machado-Cruz (1962). The presence of myxobacteria on the gills was described as were the histological changes in affected gills. The histology was similar to that described by Wood and Yasutake (1957) except that Machado-Cruz noted areas of focal necrosis on the gills. Since these trout also had a secondary fungus infection on the gills, the necrotic areas may have been caused by fungal activity. Anderson and Conroy reported bacterial gill disease in Atlantic salmon in Scotland (1969b). Ghittino (1967) described bacterial gill disease in Italy and the possible role that dried crumbled feeds may have on gill irritation leading to outbreaks of gill disease. Discussion with European fish pathologists revealed that bacterial gill disease is common in trout hatcheries but seldom described in published reports.

CONTROL

*Prevention*

*Environmental conditions.* Because poor environmental conditions appear to trigger outbreaks of bacterial gill disease, the maintenance of conditions favoring the health of salmonids is of the utmost importance. Crowding in itself may not be detrimental, but rather the increased stress from lower oxygen, accumulation of waste products, and large bacterial load resulting from crowding. An experiment designed by Davis (1946; 1953) to illustrate the effect of crowding on growth rate illustrates the above point. Fingerling rainbow trout from the same lot were placed into troughs each containing 182.3 liters (48.27 gallons) of water with a water exchange about every nine minutes. One trough received 500 fingerlings; one received 1000; one received 2000; and one received 3000. The average weight of all fish was the same as were the diet available per fish and other conditions. The experiment started March 1 and very little difference was noted in growth rate up to April 26. From that time, growth rate of trout in the larger lots was slower; on July 19 bacterial gill disease broke out in the trough with 3000 fingerlings and these trout were dropped from the experiment. While dissolved oxygen, accumulation of ammonia, and other factors detrimental to fish health were not measured, the only variable in the experiment was the number of fish, suggesting that overcrowding contributed to the outbreak of bacterial gill disease. Had the trough with 3000 fingerlings been supplied with a faster exchange of water the gill disease might not have developed.

Irritation to trout gills may contribute to the incidence and severity of bacterial gill disease. Ghittino (1967) suggested that trout feeds with large amounts of fine particulate matter may irritate gills, while inflammation of gills and epidermis of fish has been attributed to particulate matter in water (Bandt, 1959). At some hatcheries, outbreaks of gill disease often occur within twenty-four hours after a heavy rain. Particulate matter in the water plus an increase in the numbers of myxobacteria washed from soil have been suggested as triggering the outbreaks.

*Prophylactic chemotherapy.* Because salmonid culture is intensive, all outbreaks of gill disease may not be prevented by maintaining proper environmental conditions. Many hatcheries must rely on prophylactic treatments given weekly or biweekly to prevent gill disease. The following external disinfectants have been successfully used:

1. alkyl benzalkonium chloride (Roccal)
   2.0 p.p.m. of the active ingredient for one hour.

2. alkyl $C_{14}$, $C_{12}$, $C_{16}$ dimethyl benzyl ammonium chloride (Hyamine 3500)
   Same treatment as Roccal. It is good for hard water areas and is effective at water up to 550 p.p.m. total hardness.

3. pyridylmercuric acetate (PMA)

    1–2 p.p.m. for one hour. The concentration is not based on active ingredient but calculations are based on substance directly from the container.

4. Ethyl mercury phosphate (Lignasan X)

    Concentration and time of treatment same as for PMA. Also used directly from the container.

External prophylactic treatments are effective in preventing bacterial gill disease but there are limitations on their use. The availability of organic mercurials and restrictions placed on their use by health authorities severely restricts their use for control of fish diseases.

*Roccal.* (benzalkonium chlorides) This quarternary ammonium compound was introduced by Fish (1947) and has been used successfully with all species of salmonids in treating gill disease, but variations in toxicity and effectiveness were found with different batches. These variations between batches were demonstrated experimentally by Rucker (1948). In an expanded study using homologues of Roccal, it was concluded that the variable results obtained were due to the variation in the length of the carbon chain of the alkyl group (Rucker, Johnson and Ordal, 1949). The longer carbon chain homologues of Roccal were found to be more toxic to blueback salmon than the shorter ones. It was postulated that successful treatments of gill disease resulted from using the batches containing the lower chain homologue, whereas failures resulted from use of higher chain homologues. Results of the tests indicated that Roccal preparations with mixtures of the 10, 12, 14 carbon chain should offer a margin of safety between concentrations lethal to bacteria and concentrations toxic to fishes (Rucker *et al.*, 1949). Batches of Roccal used for treating salmonids should contain chiefly the 10–14 carbon chain lengths with only small amounts of the 16 and 18 carbon compounds.

*Hyamine 3500.* Experiments conducted by Warren (pers. comm., 1966) with Hyamine 3500 and Roccal have shown differences in toxicity to fishes and myxobacteria in relationship to water hardness. Rainbow trout would tolerate slightly higher concentrations of Hyamine 3500 than Roccal in very soft water whereas Hyamine was more toxic to myxobacteria in hard water than was Roccal, suggesting it would be more efficient to use this compound in areas of hard water. More experimental work is needed before a complete evaluation of this compound can be made.

*Pyridylmercuric Acetate* (Technical) (PMA). This disinfectant was suggested as a treatment for bacterial gill disease by Van Horn and Katz (1946) and tested by Rucker (1948) who found PMA effective on blueback salmon with gill disease but suggested it be tested further. This mercury compound was used widely but there were reports of toxicity to rainbow trout. The toxicity of PMA for rainbow, brook, and brown trouts was studied and results showed no toxicity to brook and brown trouts and sporadic toxicity to rainbow trout (Rogers, Hazen, Friddle and Snieszko, 1951). A relationship was noted between both the size of trout and water temperature and the toxicity of PMA for rainbows. Losses increased with a rise in water temperature and with an increase in size of the trout. It was then found that different batches of PMA varied in the contents of active ingredient (Allison, 1957) from 81.8–87.3 and batches containing more active ingredients were more toxic to rainbow trout if used at 2 or even 1 p.p.m. (it should be remembered that PMA concentrations are calculated with the substance as it comes from the container and not on the basis of active ingredient). Burrows and Palmer (1949) however found that blueback, coho, and chinook salmon, as well as steelhead and eastern brook trout, could be treated with 2 p.p.m. for one hour with no deleterious effects. This again points out the variable results obtained in regard to toxicity to rainbow trout since the steelhead trout are merely a sea-run rainbow trout. Other reports of toxicity to rainbows showed that eight-inch rainbow trout suffered mortality when treated with PMA but two-inch rainbows did not (Foster and Olsen, 1951). Also PMA was successfully used to control columnaris disease on brook, brown, and rainbow trouts during the summer but one lot of rainbow trout was lost after several treatments. Heavy rains had caused an increase in pH and decrease in water temperature which may have contributed to the increased toxicity to rainbow trout (Bryant, 1951).

In present day salmonid culture, rainbow trout may be treated up to the time they are 1–2 inches long, but this is not usually done unless other disinfectants such as Roccal do not work. Two general methods of dispensing PMA have been used. Burrows and Palmer (1949) mixed the granules directly into the pond or trough to obtain the desired concentration. They cautioned that inhalation of the fine dust from the disinfectant should be avoided and recommended the use of a respirator. To avoid the dust, Snieszko (1949) suggested that a 10% stock solution be made up from which the treatment concentration could be used. Methods of calculation of PMA solutions and treatment were also described by Snieszko (1949).

*Lignasan X*. Lignasan X, which contains ethyl mercury phosphate as the active ingredient, was found to be as effective as PMA for gill disease and more economical. The effective dose is also 2 p.p.m. and Lignasan, like PMA, is toxic to rainbow trout, even to very small (1 inch) rainbows (Rucker, Earp and Burrows, 1956). It is apparently much more toxic to myxobacteria than PMA since there is only 6.25% active ingredient compared with 83–87% active ingredient in PMA. Since Lignasan is a mercury compound it should be handled with caution.

*Treatment*

Much of the foregoing discussion on prophylactic treatments of gill disease also apply to treatment of outbreaks. The main difference is that only one application of these disinfectants is given for prophylactic treatments, whereas the procedure varies for treating epizootics. Roccal and Hyamine 3500 must be given at 1–2 p.p.m. on three consecutive days for effective treatment of an epizootic. However only one treatment of PMA or Lignasan X at 1–2 p.p.m. is usually necessary to bring an epizootic under control.

# *Fin Rot and Tail Rot*

### Definition of the Disease

Progressive erosion and disintegration of the fins of fishes is usually referred to as fin or tail rot. Although the two diseases are probably identical, it has been suggested that tail rot means caudal fin erosion and fin rot refers to erosion of other fins (Pentelow, 1947).

### Symptoms and Pathology

Development of fin and tail rot lesions in salmonid and aquarium fishes appears to be similar. The first symptom is a white line on the outer margin of the fin which progresses toward the base of the fin. As the lesion develops, the outer fin margin becomes frayed from disintegration of the soft tissues between the fin rays. The degenerative process continues until the whole fin is lost and in the case of caudal fin erosion, only a stump is left. However, if the cartilage at the base of the pectoral or pelvic fin is attacked the fin may drop off instead of eroding (Figs. 22 and 23).

Histological examination of bacterial fin rot tissue showed that the epithelial hyperplasia was probably a tissue reaction to the presence of bacteria, while the progressive destruction of the epithelium was apparently due to the lytic action of bacteria which not only attack surface tissues, but also invade connective tissues and follow the lymph channels, where the bacteria may be seen in large masses around fin rays (Davis, 1953).

Fin tissue of salmonids may also be damaged from a variety of non-infectious causes and then attacked by saprophytic water bacteria. The dorsal fin of salmonid fishes may show a thickening superficially resembling the early stage of fin rot. On close examination the edge of the fin appears smooth and lacks the ragged appearance of bacterial fin rot. The thickening is probably due to irritation resulting from crowding of the fish (Davis, 1953). Exposure to bright sunlight (containing an abundance of ultraviolet rays) may cause "sunburn" in salmonids and this may cause damage to the dorsal fin. The use of concrete raceways for propagation of salmonids often causes loss of pectoral fins from rubbing on the rough sides of the raceway (Fig. 24).

Tail rot apparently is more prevalent in marine fishes and usually involves hemorrhagic areas near the caudal fin as well as the thickening of the fin

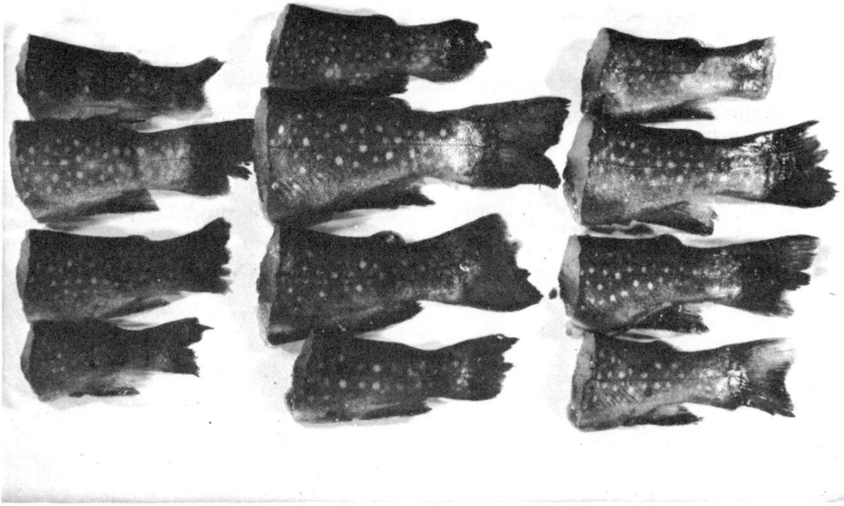

Figure 22. Caudal areas of brook trout (*Salvelinus fontinalis*) with varying intensity of tail rot. (Bullock, 1968)

Figure 23. Severe case of tail rot in goldfish (*Carassius auratus*). Fish was alive when picture was taken. Scale is in millimeters.

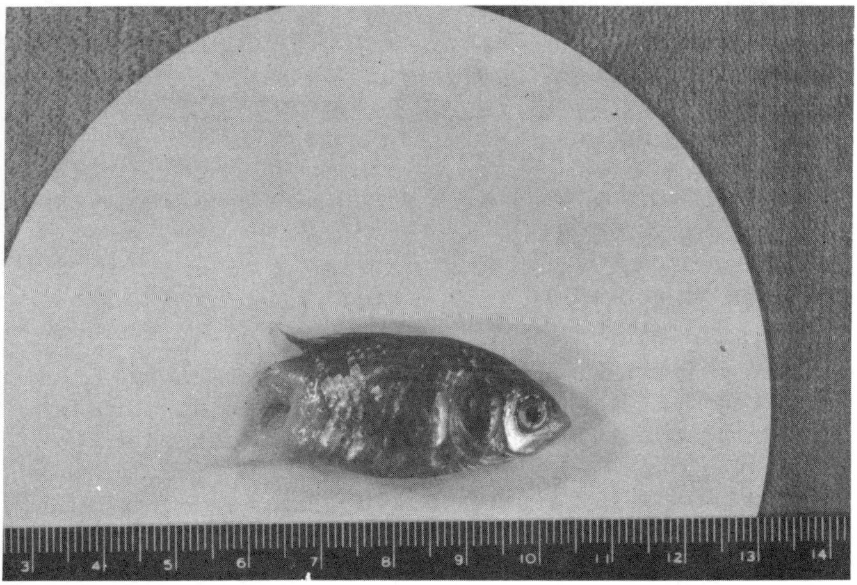

margin. It often occurs in marine fish kept in aquaria and progresses rapidly, usually causing death within a few days after gross symptoms appear (Oppenheimer, 1958; Sinderman and Rosenfield, 1954).

## Etiology

At present, it is not possible to state that a single type of bacterium is the etiologic agent of tail and fin rot. Conroy (1961a, b) found that tail rot could be experimentally produced in goldfish with *A. liquefaciens*, whereas a natural outbreak of tail rot was caused by a non-gas-producing aeromonad (*A. formicans*) with typical symptoms of the disease produced when the isolated organism was injected into healthy fish (Conroy, 1964). A fluorescent pseudomonad was isolated from a goldfish with tail rot but only transient

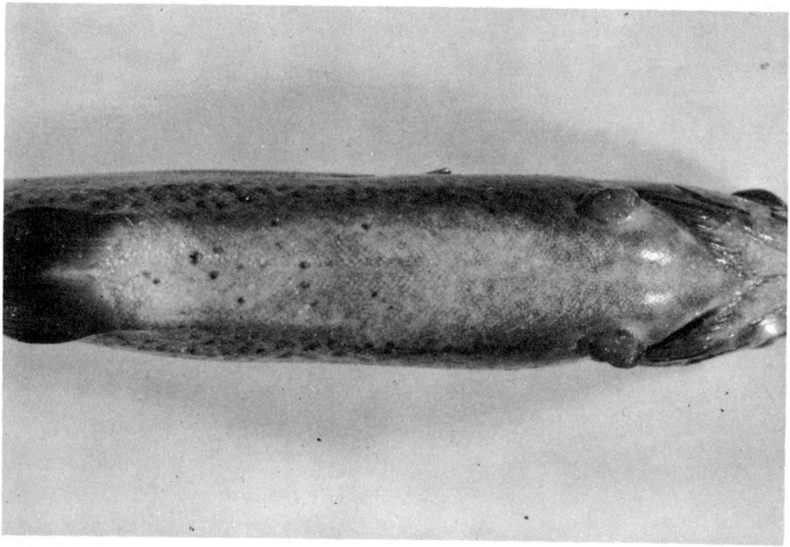

Figure 24. Loss of pectoral fins in yearling rainbow trout (*Salmo gairdneri*) from constant abrasion on sides of cement raceways.

symptoms were produced on injection of the pseudomonad into healthy fish (Conroy, 1963a). In a study of tail rot in brook trout the bacteria from tail lesions were the same types found in raceway water and they were probably acting as secondary invaders (Bullock, 1968). Undetermined species of motile, gram-negative bacteria have been isolated from cases of tail and fin rot in several species of marine fishes (Sindermann and Rosenfield, 1954; Oppenheimer, 1958). Typical symptoms of tail rot could be produced in healthy codfish (*Gadus callarias*) by injection of a pseudomonad previously isolated from codfish with tail rot (Oppenheimer, 1958).

There are at least three possibilities in regard to the etiology of fin and tail rot: 1. bacteria, usually of the *Aeromonas-Pseudomonas* group, are the direct cause; 2. these bacteria and also aquatic myxobacteria are secondary invaders which attack fins damaged by injury from crowding, scraping on concrete raceways, or other causes, such as folic acid deficiency (Halver, 1954) or an excess of Vitamin A (Poston, 1966); 3. the condition accompanies other bacterial diseases such as furunculosis, ulcer disease, and myxobacterial infections. Although fungi are not considered a cause of fin and tail rot, fishes with advanced tail or fin rot may also have super infections caused by fungi.

## Diagnosis

Diagnosis of fin and tail rot is made on the basis of the gross symptoms. A microscopic examination of stained material from affected fins will show the quantitative involvement of bacteria, and a detailed bacteriological examination of affected fins and internal organs and identification of the isolated cultures will show whether the condition was a manifestation of ulcer disease, furunculosis, a myxobacteriosis, or if it should be diagnosed as fin rot which still is a rather vague term.

## Transmission, Epizootiology, and Pathogenesis

Fin and tail rot are probably transmitted by fish to fish contact or in some cases directly from the water. Interesting observations were made by Hewitt (1937) and Connel (1937) who were able to prevent and even control fin rot in trout by disinfection of hatchery troughs with chlorine. It is also worthy to note that since wooden troughs in trout hatcheries were replaced by metal tanks, which are much easier to maintain in sanitary conditions, fin rot in trout hatcheries almost ceased to be a problem.

Fin nipping and *Gyrodactylus* instigated infections are frequently associated with fin rot (Davis, 1953) and the mechanical injury from these causes may allow secondary infection.

Pathogenesis is probably due to histolytic enzymes of invading bacteria.

## Host and Geographic Range

Fin and tail rot may affect salmonids, pondfishes, aquarium, and marine fishes. The severity of the disease may vary. For instance, in one bait-minnow hatchery in the state of Texas, 750,000 marketable minnows were lost from an epizootic of fin rot which spread from one pond to the rest of the ponds in the series (Toole and Tiller, 1964). Fin and tail rot now rarely reaches epizootic proportions in propagated salmonids. Heavily pigmented aquarium fishes such as mollies appear to be more susceptible to fin rot than lightly pigmented species (van Duijn, 1967).

The range of the disease is worldwide.

## Control Measures

*Prevention*

Since fin and tail rot are diseases caused primarily by bacteria and are aggravated by unfavorable environmental conditions and malnutrition, the best preventive measures are the maintenance of favorable environment and good sanitation. Crowding, improper temperature, deficiency of folic acid and inositol (Halver, 1954), or excess of Vitamin A (Poston, 1966) may contribute to fin rot. Even if fin rot *per se* may not cause fish losses, necrotic fins may serve as portal of entry for more virulent fish pathogens. If fin rot is a result of furunculosis, ulcer disease, or a myxobacteriosis, control measures specific for these diseases should be applied.

*Treatment*

External treatments are usually used to treat tail and fin rot; however, injection of antibiotics has also been used.

A. External treatments

1. Dipping fish in 1:2000 copper sulfate for 1–2 minutes (Davis, 1953).
2. Chlorine in form of calcium hypochlorite. Free chlorine concentration in water should not exceed 2 p.p.m. Treatment should last for 2 minutes and be stopped by neutralizing chlorine with sodium thiosulfate (Connel, 1937).
3. Dual flush treatment with 59 milliliters formalin and 59 milliliters of a 1:40 malachite green solution in approximately 113 liters (4 cu. ft.) of water (Eicher, 1947).
4. Addition of oxytetracycline (Terramycin) to aquaria water proved successful in treating warmwater fishes (Irwin, 1959). No specific dosage given, but it is assumed a concentration of 10–50 p.p.m. would be safe.
5. For aquarium species the following has been recommended (van Duijn, 1967).
   a. Phenoxethol or propylene phenoxethol 10 milliliters of a 0.1% solution per liter of aquarium water.
   b. Parachlorophenoxethol at 50 milliliters of a 0.1% solution per liter of aquarium water.

   This compound has been toxic to some species and is not recommended for general use. Also both a. and b. are given as prolonged treatments and, since they do not decompose rapidly, further additions are usually not required. Water temperature should be 15°C (60°F) or above. If no improvement in the area is noted in three days, the affected portion of the fin should be cut away.
6. Another general treatment for aquarium fishes is 100 milligrams of oxytetracycline per gallon of aquarium water each day for five days. Two drops of a 5% aqueous solution of methylene blue may be added with each treatment to control fungus (Axelrod, 1962).

Antibiotics are usually not injected or fed to propagated fishes with fin and tail rot unless ulcer disease or furunculosis is involved. With aquarium fishes or small numbers of valuable brood fish, a single intraperitoneal injection of Kanamycin at the rate of 20 milligrams per kilogram may be effective (Conroy, 1962, 1963b). The Kanamycin treatment may be combined with chloramphenicol added to the food at the rate of 1 milligram per gram of food (van Duijn, 1967).

# *Corynebacterial Diseases*

## Kidney Disease and Dee Disease

### Definition of the Disease

Diseases caused by corynebacteria have thus far been reported only in salmonids in the United States, Canada, and the British Isles. "Kidney disease" is the term used in the United States and Canada, whereas the same disease is called "Dee disease" in the British Isles (Smith, 1964). The term "Dee disease" historically preceded "kidney disease" but the latter term has been generally accepted in North America and in Europe (Reichenbach-Klinke, 1966) and will be used in this text.

### Historical

The first report on this disease appeared in the second interim report of the Furunculosis Committee (Mackie *et al.*, 1933). Typical lesions were observed in the spleen and other internal organs of the Atlantic salmon from the rivers Dee and Spey in Scotland. Disease was transmitted experimentally with tissues of diseased fish, and a small gram-positive bacillus was grown on culture media enriched with trout blood, but cultures proved avirulent for brown trout. Two years later a similar disease was reported from brook trout in a Massachusetts hatchery by Belding and Merrill (1935). The gross pathology observed was very similar to what has been observed in subsequent outbreaks of kidney disease and the bacterium was also similar except that motility was reported by Belding and Merrill (1935).

Belding and Merrill described the symptoms in detail and were also able to culture their organism on nutrient agar with the addition of defibrinated blood. Trout were experimentally infected, both with pathological material and with isolated cultures. Inflammation and necrotic lesions were produced and trout died after several weeks. Since the late 1940's, kidney disease has often been reported from cultured salmonids.

### Symptoms and Pathology

Kidney disease can best be described as a chronic disease occurring over a wide range of water temperatures. Some outbreaks begin in spring and others in the autumn months when the water temperature is declining

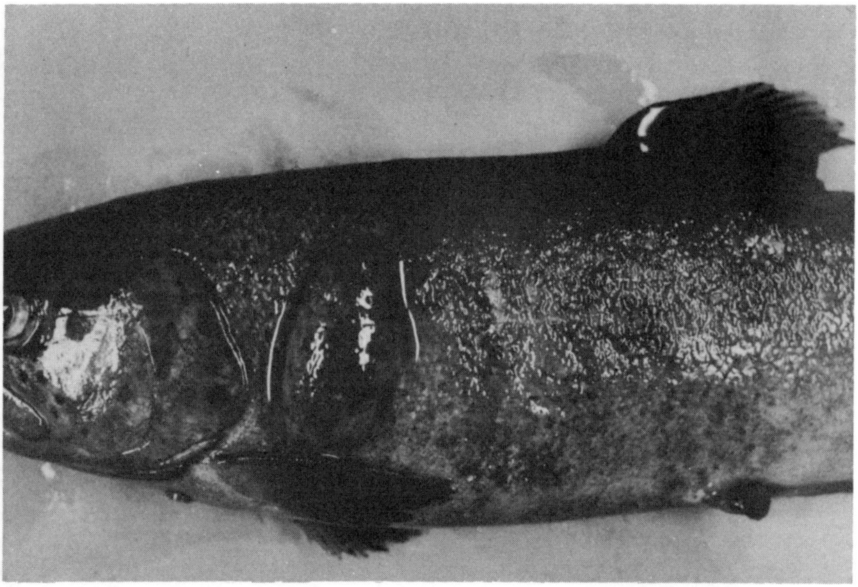

Figure 25. External symptoms of kidney disease in rainbow trout (*Salmo gairdneri*). Note the small ulcers. (This figure, reproduced in color, appears after Index.)

to 10°C or below. Mortalities during these epizootics gradually, but inevitably, increase and exact a serious toll. When epizootics occur during periods of moderate or warm temperature (13–18°C) the course of the disease may be accelerated and mortalities heavy. Detailed descriptions of the symptoms of kidney disease were given by Belding and Merrill (1935). Externally, exophthalmos was the most striking symptom and occurred in 30% of seventy-four trout examined. The exophthalmos was due to edema and serous effusion resulting from destruction of kidney tissue. Blebs and blisters were present on the sides above the lateral line (Fig. 25) and occurred in 60% of examined trout. The unruptured bleb appeared as a raised circular or elliptical area of skin, separated by fluid from the underlying tissues. Blebs varied in size from 1 to 40 millimeters and contained either a clear amber to blood-tinged fluid or purulent fluid consisting of cells, bacteria, and granular debris (Fig. 26). When muscle tissue under the bleb was invaded, it was pitted and infiltrated with a bloody, viscous, turbid fluid. On occasion, instead of superficial blebs, abscesses containing a thick, white or hemorrhagic fluid were found localized deep in muscle tissue. There was a sloughing of muscle tissue and a tendency for the fluid to spread along the intermuscular area. Hemorrhagic areas occurred along the base of the pectoral fins.

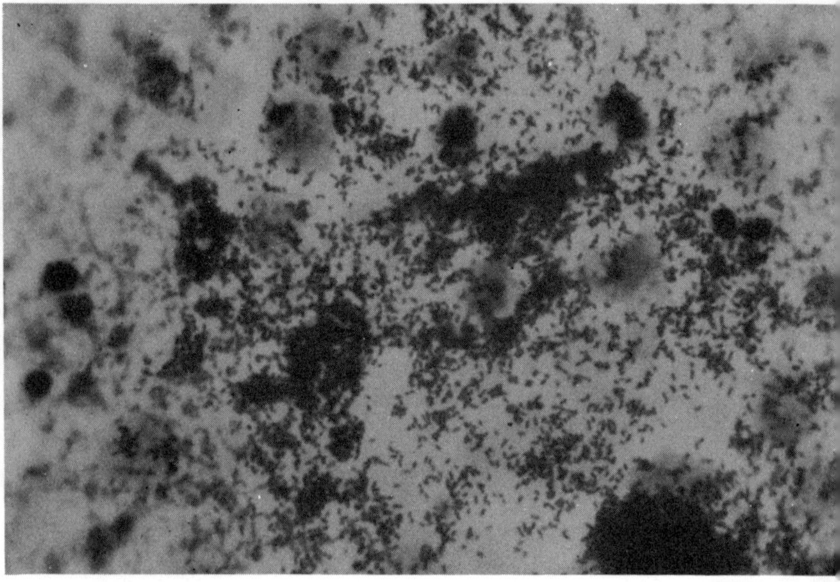

Figure 26. Photomicrograph of stained brook trout (*Salvelinus fontinalis*) kidney smear showing corynebacteria causing kidney disease (note intracellular forms. ×1000. (This figure, reproduced in color, appears after Index.)

Internally the kidneys were most frequently affected (53%). In early stages one or more greyish-white areas 2 to 5 millimeters in diameter could be observed beneath the capsule on the ventral surface (Figs. 27 and 28). These usually contained a thick, white, finely-granular fluid consisting of cells, leucocytes, bacteria, and cell debris. Occasionally the white areas were firm and friable. As the disease progresses, the number and size of the areas increase. Authors believed that the areas in resistant trout had time to coalesce into large greyish-white masses. In such cases the kidney was usually consistently swollen. About one-third of the trout had an accumulation of clear amber or hemorrhagic, peritoneal fluid; whereas, one-fourth had pericardial erosions, with nearly all cases showing some stage of pericarditis. Abscesses occurred in the livers in slightly over one-fifth of the trout. Typically they occurred on the ventral side and were of pinpoint size.

Usually there was no gross pathology in the spleen except for an apparent increase in size. Less than one-tenth of the examined trout had minute abscesses. Fifteen percent of affected trout had hemorrhagic areas in the reproductive organs. In some cases small abscesses similar to the ones observed in the liver were seen in the testes but were uncommon in the

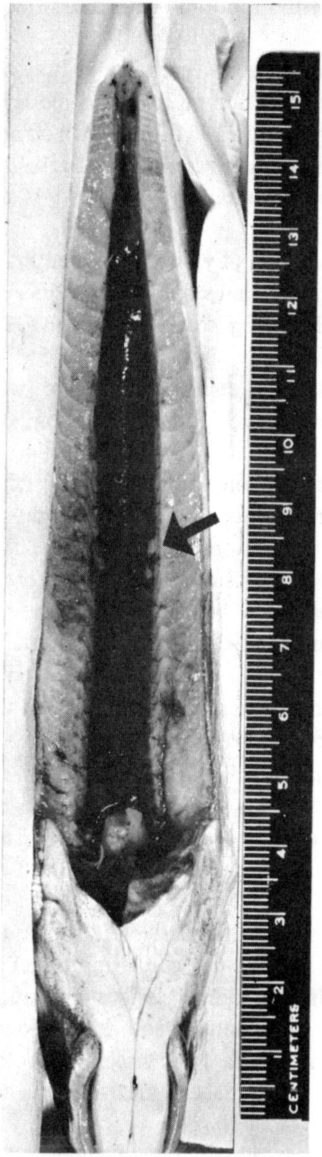


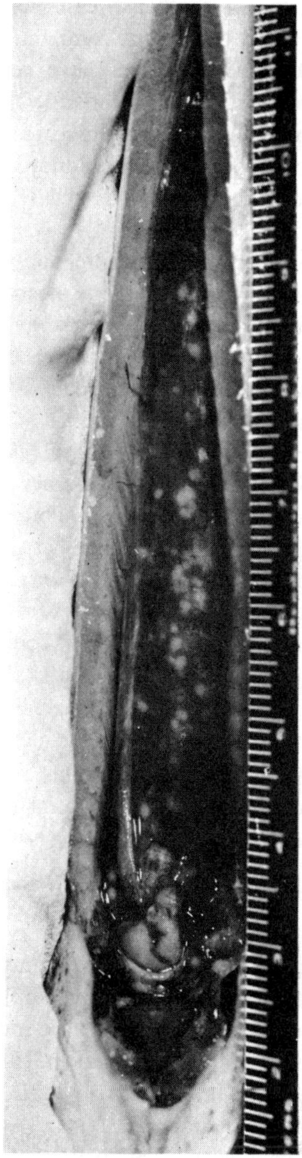

Figure 27. Exposed kidney of healthy male pink salmon (*Oncorhynchus gorbuscha*). Arrow shows corpuscle of Stannius.

Figure 28. Exposed kidney of male pink salmon (*Oncorhynchus gorbuscha*) with kidney disease. Note the numerous lesions through the kidney. (Courtesy of Dr. Gordon Bell)

ovaries. As in other diseases, congestion of the hind gut with distention of the blood vessels was common.

Other investigators have reported similar gross pathology; however, among salmon in Scotland, the most common symptom was petechial hemorrhages of the peritoneal muscle lining (Smith, 1964). Also with chinook salmon fingerlings, the kidney is the prime organ affected, whereas the liver is most frequently affected in adult chinook salmon (Wood and Wallis, 1955).

An interesting phenomenon was the formation of white, false membranes which covered the liver, spleen, gonads, and at times the swim bladder and peritoneal muscle (Snieszko and Griffin, 1955; Smith, 1964). Smith (1964) has associated the appearance of the false membranes with the water temperature in that Scottish salmon develop the membrane at water temperatures below 8.3°C (47°F), whereas infected salmon show only necrotic lesions above 9.4°C (49°F).

Kidney disease and another (non-infectious) condition known as visceral granuloma may occur simultaneously in brook trout, and it was thought that a relationship might exist between the two conditions. Further examination of the two diseases has shown that they are distinct and their occurrence together was coincidental (Wood and Yasutake, 1956b). Histological description of kidney disease by Wood and Yasutake (1956c) was complicated by the presence of granuloma in these trout. The two diseases were described as if the histological changes were due only to kidney disease. When described separately, the histological picture of the two conditions is very different. Granuloma will be discussed more fully in another chapter. A brief description of visceral granuloma and its differences from kidney disease are given since the gross appearance of diseased kidney lesions caused by kidney disease and visceral granuloma are superficially similar and may be confused.

In salmonid fishes with typical bacterial kidney disease, the kidney lesions, if present, are soft and contain a greyish pus consisting of cellular debris and gram-positive diplobacilli. If the kidney lesions are due to visceral granuloma they are much harder and compact and do not contain the kidney disease organism. However, kidney disease and visceral granuloma may exist simultaneously in the same fish which makes a clear-cut diagnosis rather difficult.

Histological examination of salmon with kidney disease showed focal necrosis in the spleen and liver with the bacteria occurring on the periphery of the lesion and tissue debris in the center. Giant cell formation was not observed. Kidney sections showed necrotic areas but the causative organism was much more often found in large numbers in tissue surrounding the renal tubules (Smith, 1964).

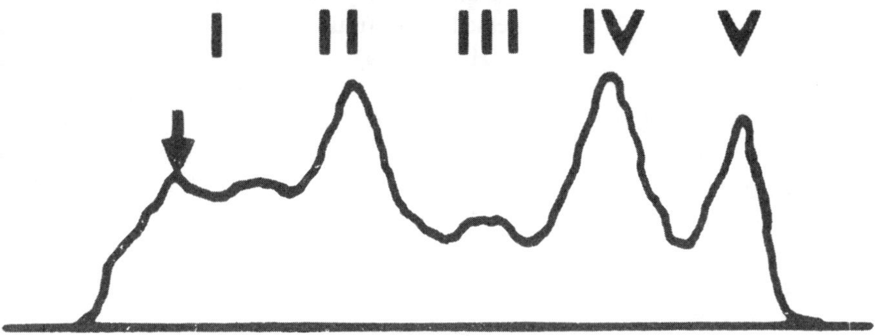


Figure 29. Electrophorogram of plasma proteins from a normal male brook trout. Arrow indicates point of application. (Hunn, 1964)

Because of the massive destruction of various tissues it was postulated that significant changes should occur in physiologic parameters associated with hematopoietic, liver and kidney function (Hunn, 1964). Yearling brook trout with chronic kidney disease were examined with respect to hematocrit, total protein, and electrophoretic pattern of their sera. In infected trout, the hematocrit was reduced by 14% compared to non-infected trout, whereas total plasma protein dropped 52% (Table 12). Electrophoretic analysis of the plasma proteins indicated that the faster migrating albumin fractions (IV and V) (Figs. 29 and 30) were reduced in infected trout. There was also an observed difference in susceptibility between males and females.

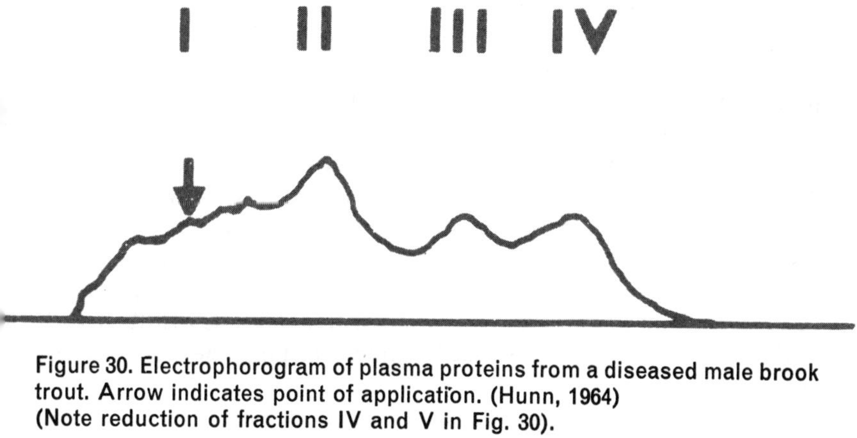


Figure 30. Electrophorogram of plasma proteins from a diseased male brook trout. Arrow indicates point of application. (Hunn, 1964)
(Note reduction of fractions IV and V in Fig. 30).

TABLE 12. Hematocrit and total plasma protein values for normal and diseased brook trout.
(Hunn, 1964)

| *No. of Fish* | *Type of fish* | *Parameter* | *Mean* ± S.E. | *Range* |
|---|---|---|---|---|
| | | Normal trout | | |
| 114 | Both sexes | Hematocrit | 39 ±1 | 19 –51 |
| 67 | Males | Total plasma protein, g% | 4.5±0.1 | 3.0– 6.0 |
| 52 | Females | *Idem* | 4.6±0.1 | 3.0– 7.4 |
| 21 | Normal females resorbing eggs | ,, | 5.9±0.4 | 3.8–11.0 |
| | | Diseased trout | | |
| 34 | Both sexes | Hematocrit | 22 ±1 | 7 –40 |
| 26 | Males | Total plasma protein, g% | 2.2±0.2 | 1.0– 4.2 |
| 7 | Females | *Idem* | 2.2±0.2 | 1.4– 3.2 |
| 5 | Females resorbing eggs | ,, | 2.7±0.6 | 1.4– 4.4 |

## Etiology

The causative agent of kidney disease is a small (0.3–0.5μ × 0.5–1.0μ) non-motile, non-acid-fast, gram-positive diplobacillus. This organism is difficult to grow. It was grown successfully in chick embryo tissues (Earp, Ellis and Ordal, 1953). Now a medium containing cycteine-hydrochloride and human blood is used (Ordal and Earp, 1956).

A gram-positive diplobacillus was isolated from trout by Belding and Merrill (1935) and also from salmon during the early outbreaks reported by the Furunculosis Committee (Mackie *et al.*, 1935). However, in the light of present knowledge, it is possible that in neither instance was the specific corynebacterium of kidney disease isolated. For example, the organism in the Furunculosis Committee report could not be experimentally proved pathogenic. Also the organism isolated from trout by Belding and Merrill (1935) differed in several characteristics from present day descriptions. These workers reported their isolate was 1–4μ long, grew feebly at 37°C, was motile, and reached a colony size of 0.5 millimeters in forty-eight hours. The most recent characterization of strains from authentic cases of kidney disease indicate the organism is at most 1.5μ long, is non-motile, does not grow at 37°C, and usually requires at least a week for visible growth to occur (Ordal and Earp, 1956; Smith, 1964). It is probable that these early workers were working with a mixed culture containing the kidney disease organism.

At present the bacterium is classified as an unspeciated *Corynebacterium.*

## Diagnosis

Observance of the external and internal symptoms just described, and the presence of a gram-positive diplobacillus, usually constitutes adequate diagnosis of kidney disease. This method is not definitive in the sense of actually identifying the organism of kidney disease, but because the coryne-bacterium grows slowly, this serves as a practical diagnostic procedure for the present. However it should be pointed out that since kidney disease is chronic and other diseases such as furunculosis may occur simultaneously, presence of low numbers of the kidney disease organism in sick fishes may not mean the fishes are dying from this disease and attempts should be made to diagnose the presence of other diseases. If salmonids are dying from kidney disease, the bacterium should be present in the tissues in very great numbers.

Again it should be emphasized that kidney disease and visceral granuloma often occur together, particularly in brook trout, and one should be careful not to confuse these diseases.

Another precaution should also be taken in the diagnosis of bacterial kidney disease. The melanin pigment granules are often present in large numbers in the smears made from kidney, liver, or spleen of fishes. They are of the same size as the kidney disease organism and separation of these two in gram-stained smears requires considerable experience. In smears stained with methylene blue, the kidney disease organism stains blue while pigment granules remain brown-black. In unstained control smears, pigment granules are also brown-black while the bacteria remain almost invisible.

## Transmission and Pathogenesis

The mode of transmission of kidney disease among hatchery stocks has not been unequivocally established; there are, however, several likely explanations of the mode of transmission. There is circumstantial evidence for transmission on or in the fertilized egg. Also the occurrence of parasites on or in fishes with kidney disease suggests that the parasites may introduce the disease or lower the resistance of the fishes to infection (Wood and Yasutake, 1956a). In the western United States experimental transmission was accomplished by feeding infected salmon viscera to fingerling chinook salmon held at 12.8°C (55°F) (Wood and Wallis, 1955). In the eastern United States, experimental infections were difficult to establish. Attempts to transmit the disease to brook trout by feeding were unsuccessful (Snieszko and Griffin, 1955; Wolf and Dunbar, 1959). In fact feeding bile salts or glass shards along with bacteria-laden food to brook trout also failed to produce infection (Wolf and Dunbar, 1959). Experimental infection of the same lot of brook trout was accomplished by abrasion of the skin followed by exposure to the bacterium. This was accomplished by allowing trout to abrade themselves on bricks placed in tanks followed by addition of bacteria to the water, or manually abrading the skin of trout with garnet abrasive paper dipped into a suspension of bacteria. However, forty-eight days elapsed before the first mortality occurred (Wolf and Dunbar, 1959). Therefore at least for brook trout, it is likely that the portal of entry of the kidney disease organism is through skin which has been punctured by parasites or mechanical factors (Wolf and Dunbar, 1959). As with many bacterial infections, temperature of the water affected the disease course and greater losses from kidney disease were obtained at 7°C (45°F) than at 13°C (54°F). Also the strain isolated from trout was more virulent than the one isolated from pacific salmon.

Finally in hatcheries with a water supply containing fishes the disease may be transmitted from infected feral fishes.

The occurrence of kidney disease is probably significantly affected by environmental conditions which may explain its occurrence at particular trout hatcheries. At one time this disease was a problem only in those regions which bordered on the sea, however the range has been extended with the finding of the disease in hatcheries in inland states. This put an end to the belief that the incidence was associated with proximity to the sea and possibly transmitted by raw marine fish used as feed (Wolf, 1956). Other environmental factors, notably water chemistry, seemed to affect the disease incidence in that kidney disease was most severe at hatcheries with soft water (Warren, 1963a). A study was undertaken to examine this phenomenon at hatcheries throughout the United States and it was found that as the hardness of the water decreased the severity of kidney disease increased. The extent of this relationship is not known and other factors may be involved. For example, postulated vectors of the disease such as parasites may flourish in soft stream water and be absent in hard spring water. Also the disease-resistance mechanism of the salmonids may be influenced by water chemistry (Warren, 1963a). However, the relationship between disease incidence and water chemistry is important and hopefully more experimental work will be done on this subject.

Although the actual mode of pathogenesis of the bacterium is not known, the chronic nature of the disease and the massive tissue destruction leave little doubt that the cause of death is destruction of the function of vital organs (Wood and Yasutake, 1956c) with resulting anemia and other changes in blood chemistry already discussed (Hunn, 1964).

## Host and Geographic Range

Pacific chinook, coho, and sockeye salmons are the most susceptible, with infection occurring before the fingerlings migrate to the open sea. Kidney disease also occurs in pink salmon (*O. gorbuscha*) (Bell, 1961) and steelhead trout (Earp *et al.*, 1953). Of the three main species of trouts, the brook trout are most susceptible; brown trout are intermediate, and rainbow are most resistant. Lake trout (*S. namaycush*), cutthroat trout (*S. clarki*), and Atlantic salmon (*S. salar*) are also susceptible. Occurrence of kidney disease among non-salmonids as far as the authors know is unknown.

The reported geographic range at present is limited to North America and the British Isles.

## Control

Effective control of kidney disease depends upon knowledge of the sources and modes of infection, which is incomplete at the present. Since egg transmission is a possibility, eggs should be obtained from parents free of the disease. Also since feeding of infected viscera transmitted the disease to fingerling Pacific salmon (Wood and Wallis, 1955), this practice has been abandoned or the viscera pasteurized before being fed. At hatcheries where the disease does not occur, the best control measure is to prevent kidney disease from being introduced; at hatcheries where the disease does occur, steps should be taken to minimize its spread. Such practices as strict quarantine or antiseptic disposal of infected lots of fish, and disinfection of all facilities and equipment will help to prevent the spread of kidney disease.

Prophylactic chemotherapy has been recommended (Wood and Wallis, 1955) and used with salmon where the disease is an annual problem. Sulfamethazine and more recently sulfamerazine have been used at the rate of 4.2 grams per 100 kilograms of salmon per day and fed to the salmon from the time they start feeding until they are released to the sea. Although the probability of selecting sulfa-resistant strains of the kidney disease bacterium seemed likely, none has so far been reported and prophylactic chemotherapy is still being used.

### CHEMOTHERAPY

Kidney disease is one of the most difficult of the bacterial diseases to treat, probably because of its chronic nature and also because bacteria may occur intracellularly. A number of sulfonamides alone or in combination were used to control kidney disease. Sulfadiazine was fed to infected fingerling salmon at the rate of 25 grams per 100 kilograms of fish per day for seven days then 13 grams per 100 kilograms of fish per day for twenty-one days. During the first half of the following month fish were not treated, then were treated at the 13 grams level for the remainder of the month (Rucker, Bernier, Whipple, and Burrows, 1951). Brook trout were treated with sulfamerazine alone or in combination with sulfadiazine and/or sulfaguanidine. Treatment lasted for twenty-nine days and trout basically received 25 grams per 100 kilograms of fish per day (Allison, 1958). Snieszko and Griffin (1955) recommended either sulfisoxazole, sulfamerazine, or sulfamethazine be used at the 16 to 20 grams per 100 kilograms of fish per day level until mortality is reduced and then weekly (or shorter) periods of drug feeding be given during the months kidney disease is a problem. In all the treatments with sulfonamides, only temporary control was usually achieved with mortalities again occurring after treatment was stopped.

Wolf and Dunbar (1959) tested thirty-four therapeutic agents *in vitro* against the kidney disease bacterium and from the results obtained they selected eleven of the drugs for *in vivo* trials. Results from the *in vivo* trials indicated that erythromycin was the drug of choice. A treatment of 9–10 grams per 100 kilograms of trout per day for three weeks was found to give good but not always complete control. Another form of erythromycin (erythromycin thiocyanate) has been used with success to control kidney disease but some toxic effects, including extreme nervousness, were noted (Piper, 1961). An attempt was made to reproduce experimentally the toxic effects. However, in order to show toxicity from erythromycin thiocyanate it was necessary to use five times the recommended treatment level of the drug (Warren, 1963b). Present recommendations are for erythromycin U.S.P. at 9–10 grams per 100 kilograms of fish per day for three weeks.

## Other Corynebacterial Diseases

Recently a bacterium was isolated from diseased salmon in Britain which, although apparently a *Corynebacterium* sp., differed from the kidney disease bacterium (Ajmal and Hobbs, 1967). Unlike the kidney disease bacterium, this organism is 2.0–2.5μ long and attacks carbohydrates, producing acid but no gas. However, symptoms and gross pathology of the infected salmon was similar to that produced by the kidney disease bacterium. Attempts to infect goldfish with either macerated, whole, infected kidney or kidney filtrate were unsuccessful (Ajmal and Hobbs, 1967).

# *Mycobacterial, Nocardial and Streptomyces Diseases*

## Introduction

Bacteria belonging to the genera *Mycobacterium* and *Nocardia* which possess the property of acid-fastness cause diseases in a wide variety of freshwater, marine, and aquarium fishes, although fish pathogenic mycobacteria are much better known. A recent publication (Heuschmann-Brunner, 1965) pointed out that nocardial infections have been observed in six species of fishes and emphasized the need for careful identification of acid-fast bacteria. Inter-relationships do exist among the *Mycobacteria* and *Nocardiae* in that (based on phage susceptibility) the *Streptomycetes* and mycobacteria are joined through the *Nocardiae* (Manion, Bradley, Zinneman and Hall, 1964). The majority of this section will, however, be devoted to mycobacterial infections.

## Definition of the Disease

As a rule most mycobacterial infections in fishes have been referred to as fish tuberculosis or piscine tuberculosis. This usage has been challenged and it has been suggested that the more general term fish mycobacteriosis be used instead (Parisot and Wood, 1966). Although the use of the term fish tuberculosis is warranted because the pathology is similar to tuberculosis in warm-blooded animals, there are differences in pathological changes; with infections of cold-blooded vertebrates there is usually a weak inflammatory response and an absence of giant cells, whereas these changes are typical in tuberculosis in warm-blooded animals. Also there are differences among the mycobacterial species which cause diseases in warm-blooded and cold-blooded animals. For example, mycobacteria from fishes and human beings have different staining characteristics in infected tissues (Parisot and Decker, 1960). Finally, there are at present three recognized species pathogenic for fishes. For these reasons, fish mycobacteriosis seems more descriptive and will be used throughout the discussion.

## Historical

The first description of a mycobacterial infection in fish was in 1897 (Bataillon, Dubard, and Terre, 1897) and concerned carp in a pond in France contaminated with sputa and excreta from tuberculous persons. The carp developed a small gray lesion between the abdominal wall and ovary which was shown, when excised and examined histologically, to be a tubercule containing acid-fast bacilli. The organism was pathogenic for frogs and lizards but not for pigeons or guinea pigs. Attempts were subsequently made to determine the incidence of infections by acid-fast bacilli in marine fishes taken on the high seas, examination of fishes brought into several markets revealed no infections, and it was concluded that such infections are rare (Bertarelli and Bucchia, 1910). However, in 1913 a spontaneous mycobacterial infection was reported in cod (Johnstone, 1913; Alexander, 1913) and since that time infections in many species of marine, anadromous, aquarium, and freshwater fishes have been observed.

## Symptoms and Pathology

The symptoms produced by mycobacterial infections vary depending on the types of fishes affected. For example, in fishes maintained in aquaria the main symptoms may be: 1. emaciation; 2. loss of appetite; 3. loss of color; 4. scale defects and loss of scales, fin destruction; 5. exopthalmia; 6. deformities of the jaw and vertebrae. The fish may become apathetic and remain in the corner of the aquarium or swim in jerky motion (Amlacher, 1961). The most characteristic symptom in the neon tetra is a yellowish discoloration of the normally brilliant red markings on the side of the body (Axelrod, 1962; Nigrelli and Vogel, 1963). Ulcerous lesions on the mouth and dorsal fin were reported in the three spot gourami (*Trichogaster trichopterus*) and pearl gourami (*T. leeri*) (Conroy and Valdez, 1964; Conroy, 1963c).

Among the susceptible anadromous fishes, external symptoms may be absent but some affected fishes may show one or more of the symptoms: 1. a stunted appearance; 2. a brighter than normal color; 3. lack of development of secondary sexual characteristics (Parisot, 1958).

Gross internal pathology among all affected species is fairly similar. Discrete gray-white miliary lesions, or at times necrotic lesions, may be present in the liver and sometimes in the kidney and spleen (Parisot, 1958; Wood and Ordal, 1958; Nigrelli and Vogel, 1963). With infected fishes, acid-fast bacilli may be seen in stained smears from the gills, heart, musculature, pyloric caeca, skin lesions, eyes, brain, gonads, and messenteries (Nigrelli and Vogel, 1963; Wood and Ordal, 1958). With salmonids, liver tissue may be almost completely replaced with acid-fast bacilli (Parisot, 1958). Visceral adhesions are a common occurrence in both aquarium and salmonid fishes (Wood and Ordal, 1958; Nigrelli and Vogel, 1963).

Histopathologically, mycobacterial lesions in fishes resemble the tubercular lesions in warm-blooded animals except that there is a milder or no inflammatory response, an absence of typical giant cells, and little or no caseation (Nigrelli and Vogel, 1963). With stained sections containing lesions, the acid-fast organisms appear mostly in the center of the lesions.

The lesions become necrotic and in time structures known as "yellow bodies" appear (Jahnel, 1940). Histological sections showing advanced disease wherein lesions have fused are similar to what is seen in *Ichthyosporidium* granulomas (Amlacher, 1961). Histological examination of nodules from several types of marine fishes with mycobacterial infections showed the nodules were granulomas with acid-fast bacteria occurring in and around the monocytes (Sato, 1962). Two types of granulomatous nodules were observed in these fishes; one was a slowly developing lesion composed of epitheloid cells with a wall of fibroblasts, and the second was a rapidly produced lesion containing numerous histocytes filled with acid-fast bacilli (Sato, 1963).

## Etiology

The mycobacteria from fishes are gram-positive, acid-fast (Fig. 31), non-motile rods, generally 1–4μ long by 0.3–0.7μ wide although the length of some strains has been given as up to 12μ. It is possible that acid-fast bacteria other than mycobacteria were mistakenly included which would account for the variable lengths. Several mycobacteria have been described from fishes in different types of environment and these species are discussed below.

Figure 31. Acid fast stain of chinook salmon (*Oncorhynchus tshawytscha*) gill tissue showing mycobacteria. (This figure, reproduced in color, appears after Index.)

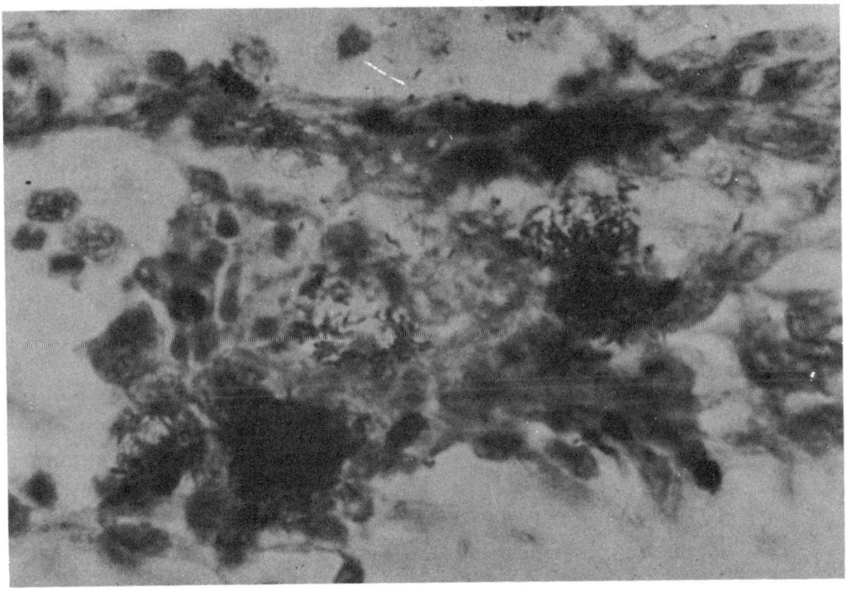

1. *M. piscium.* This was the first species described. It was isolated from carp and described in 1902 (Bataillon, Moeller and Terre, 1902), and it produced experimental infections in frogs and lizards but not in warm-blooded animals.
2. *M. marinum.* This species was the first described mycobacterium from marine fish and was isolated from Atlantic croakers (*Micropogon undulatus*), sergeant majors (*Abudefduf mauritii*), and sea bass (*Centropristes striatus L.*) in the Philadelphia Aquarium (Aronson, 1926).
3. *M. platypoecilus.* This mycobacterium was isolated from the freshwater Mexican fighting fish (*Platypoecilus maculatus*) and described by Baker and Hagen (1942).
4. *M. anabanti.* The Siamese fighting fish (*Macropodus opercularis*) was the source of this isolate and it was described by Besse (1949).
5. *M. fortuitum Cruz.* This mycobacterium was originally isolated from a cold abscess in a human being and described by Cruz (1938). Mycobacterial isolates from a neon tetra (*Hyphessobrycon innesi*) from the New York Aquarium (Nigrelli, 1953) were found to fit the species description of *M. fortuitum* and represented the first occurrence of this mycobacterium in freshwater fish (Ross and Broncato, 1959).
6. *M. salmoniphilum* sp. nov. Strains of this acid-fast bacillus were isolated from the kidneys of salmon and although the isolates were similar to *M. fortuitum* they appeared to differ in enough characteristics to be considered a separate species (Ross, 1960).
7. *Mycobacterium balnei.* This mycobacterium was isolated from skin lesions of persons swimming in cement swimming pools and also from the water and sides of the pool. Two cases of skin granulomas in human beings caused by *M. balnei* were recorded with the granulomas developing from abrasions received from a fish tank (Swift and Cohen, 1962). This species is thought to be closely related to *M. marinum* (Bojalil, Cerbon and Trujillo, 1962) and also *M. platypoecilus* (Shaffer and Davis, 1961).

Of the above species, only *M. marinum*, *M. platypoecilus*, and *M. fortuitum* are recognized in the seventh edition of *Bergey's Manual of Determinative Bacteriology* (Breed *et al.*, 1957).

## Diagnosis

Accurate diagnosis of a mycobacterial infection is accomplished by first performing an acid-fast stain on a smear from kidney, spleen, or other affected organs and then demonstrating that the bacterium is a mycobacterium and not another acid-fast species such as *Nocardia.* To determine if the isolated bacterium is a mycobacterium requires performance of diagnostic tests described in *Identification of Fish Pathogenic Bacteria.*

## Transmission, Epizootiology, and Pathogenesis

The natural mode of infection is generally conceded to be from ingestion of the organism (Nigrelli and Vogel, 1963) and, in the case of propagated salmonids, from the practice of feeding raw contaminated salmon viscera (Wood and Ordal, 1958). Transmission by transovarian passage is considered a definite possibility in viviparous fishes (Nigrelli and Vogel, 1963) but could not be shown for oviparous fishes (Ross and Johnson, 1962). Further evidence to support the theory of transovarian transmission was obtained by Conroy (1965, 1966a) with regards to a spontaneous outbreak of the disease in platies in Argentina. Of several specimens received for examination, one proved to be a gravid female. On autopsy, seven quite mature embryos were detected in the ovary, which organ was seen to be contaminated by acid-fast bacteria. Histological studies of these embryos revealed the presence of acid-fast bacteria within the embryonic tissues themselves, situated in a position corresponding to the pharyngeo-oesophagal region. It is interesting to note that an unnamed mycobacterium was isolated and found to be pathogenic for freshwater snails in the family Planorbidae. During attempts to infect snails it was found that no differences were noted among controls and infected snails with regard to growth, fecundity, or feeding, and mortalities could not directly be attributed to the mycobacterium (Michelson, 1961). Although attempts to infect fishes were not tried, it is possible that the snails were carriers of the mycobacterium and could transmit the organism to fishes.

Although it is difficult to precisely define various disease terms, fish mycobacteriosis tends to be more of a chronic than an acute disease, although it progresses faster in some aquarium species. Once established, the mycobacteria produce necrotic lesions in major organs such as the liver or spleen and impair the function of the organ, which results in death of the fish (Amlacher, 1961).

The discovery of a tuberculosis-like infection in cold-blooded vertebrates has given rise to much controversy as to whether these mycobacteria are capable of producing tuberculosis in warm-blooded vertebrates, and also whether mycobacteria from homiotherms can produce infections in cold-blooded animals.

Bataillon and his colleagues believed that the carp which they examined had been infected from human tubercle bacilli, present in the feces and sputa of a tuberculous human subject and had found their way into the water in which the fish were living. Bataillon and Terre (1897) and Terre (1902) conducted a number of studies with a view to determining whether their isolate was of piscine or human origin, and they concluded that the human tubercle bacillus may become adapted to fishes. They further suggested that the piscine bacillus is capable of producing a tubercular infection in warm-blooded animals, even though their results were not very conclusive on this point. Bataillon *et al.*, (1897) also claimed to have adapted this strain to a warm-blooded host, though it has since been suggested by Valtis (1932) that the carp may have been infected by the piscine variety and simultaneously housed the human bacillus.

The interest aroused by these claims may be seen from the large number of published papers supporting refutation of the views of Bataillon, Dubard, and Terre (1897). Anche and Hobbs (1897) showed that frogs may present lesions similar to those resulting from the action of live tubercle bacilli on inoculation of dead bacilli into the peritoneal cavity. Other authors who denied the possibility of an adaptation of the cold-blooded type to a warm-blooded host include Nicolas and Lesieur (1899), Lubarsch (1900), Sion (1900), and Herr (1901).

Recent experimentation has indicated that by temperature manipulation mycobacteria from cold-blooded vertebrates can be adapted to grow in certain body areas of warm-blooded animals and that mycobacteria from warm-blooded animals can be grown in cold-blooded animals. For example, *M. leprae* apparently multiplied when injected into perch (Chaussihand and Besse, 1951) and *M. marinum* has produced infections in warm-blooded animals when injected into the extremities, which had a lower temperature than the main body (Clark and Shepard, 1963). While progress is being made on the question of adaptation of mycobacteria from homoiotherms and poikilotherms, the limits of such adaptation are not yet known.

## Host and Geographic Range

The number of fishes susceptible to mycobacterial infections is large; one publication reports 120 susceptible species belonging to 84 genera, 34 families, and 10 orders (Vogel, 1958). The most susceptible species occur in the families Characinidae, Cyprinidae, Poecilidae, Cichlidae (Nigrelli and Vogel, 1963; Amlacher, 1961), and Salmonidae (Wood and Ordal, 1958; Parisot, 1958). The disease has been of economic importance in the anadromous fishes since many infected salmon often would not live long enough to be spawned. More detailed information concerning the genus and species of affected fishes can be obtained from Amlacher (1961), Nigrelli and Vogel (1963), and Lucky and Vanek (1962).

As might be expected from the number of affected fishes the occurrence of the disease is worldwide.

## Control

### PREVENTION

Since no standard treatment of mycobacterial fish infections exists, prevention is the only means of effectively controlling the disease. Although the end results are the same, the methods used to prevent mycobacterial infection in aquarium and hatchery fishes differ. With aquarium fishes, the maintenance of strict sanitation in aquaria is of utmost importance. Also avoidance of crowding the fishes is important. Five liters of water for each fish has been recommended (Amlacher, 1961). If new fishes are added to the aquaria, they should be visually examined for signs of the disease and should always be quarantined for two to four weeks before being placed with the other fishes.

The prevention of mycobacterial infections in propagated Pacific salmon is entirely different and clearly demonstrates how manipulation of hatchery practices can greatly reduce certain diseases. Mycobacteriosis in salmon was first observed in 1952 among adult chinook salmon returning from the sea (Wood and Ordal, 1958). The fish had been routinely examined to detect the presence of corynebacterial kidney disease. Kidney disease bacteria were absent but gram-positive and acid-fast organisms were found in large numbers. To determine the incidence, range, and significance of this disease, studies involving several species of returning salmon were undertaken. During the next several years, microscopic examination of acid-fast stained smears from the liver and other viscera of salmon returning to federal and state hatcheries in the states of Washington, Oregon, and California, revealed an incidence of from 0–21% infection with one lot of ten abnormal salmon showing nine infected fish (Table 13) (Ross, Earp and Wood, 1959). The incidence of the disease among marked hatchery fish rose from year to year in many areas and the practice of feeding raw salmon viscera to the young hatchery fish was incriminated. The viscera taken from infected adult salmon and fed to young salmon was thought to be the major source of the contamination (Wood and Ordal, 1958; Ross *et al.*, 1959). Although clinically the disease was only seen in returning adults the methods used to detect acid-fast bacteria may not have been suitable for demonstrating the organisms in the young salmon going to

TABLE 13. Percent of acid-fast bacilli infections in adult fish returning to federal hatcheries in Washington, Oregon, and California. (Ross, Earp and Wood, 1959). (1957 Return).

| *Hatchery* | | *Total No. examined* | *Total No. infected* | *Percent infected* |
|---|---|---|---|---|
| Coleman, Calif. | fall and spring chinook | 93 | 20 | 21.5 |
| Eagle Creek, Ore. | steelhead | 22 | 0 | 0.0 |
| Quilcene, Wash. | silvers | 85 | 1 | 1.1 |
| Leavenworth, Wash. | sockeye | 117 | 0 | 0.0 |
| Winthrop, Wash. | summer chinook | 31 | 0 | 0.0 |
| | sockeye | 107 | 1 | 0.9 |
| Spring Creek, Wash. | fall chinook | 300 | 7 | 2.3 |
| *Abnormal* | | | | |
| Spring Creek, Wash. | fall chinook | 10 | 9 | 90.0 |

sea. Supporting the theory of infection by feeding infected viscera was the observation that salmon free from acid-fast bacilli were found only in hatcheries where raw salmon viscera was never fed to the fish (Ross, 1963). However, in a lake in Idaho apparently supporting only wild populations of salmon, two of 368 salmon were infected with acid-fast bacilli (Ross *et al.*, 1959). The disease is also rare in wild salmon (Table 14) in areas where they were not exposed to released hatchery fish (Ross *et al.*, 1959; Wood and Ordal, 1958). Since the practice of feeding raw infected salmon viscera has been discontinued the incidence of mycobacteriosis has been greatly reduced.

#### CHEMOTHERAPY

There is no established effective treatment for mycobacterial infection among aquarium or hatchery fishes. *In vitro* tests have shown mycobacteria from fish to be sensitive to Kanamycin (Conroy and Solarolo, 1965) and an infection in Mexican platyfish was apparently treated successfully by incorporating Kanamycin in the food at the rate of 10 mg percent. No acid-fast bacteria were observed after three to four days of treatment (Conroy, 1966b).

TABLE 14. Incidence of tuberculosis in wild and hatchery fish, 1956. (Wood and Ordal, 1958)

| *Location* | *Species* | *No. of fish examined* | *No of tuberculous fish* |
|---|---|---|---|
| Wild Fish | | | |
| Little Nestucca River | Chum (Adults) | 6 | 0 |
| Nestucca River | Chum ,, | 8 | 0 |
| Whiskey Creek | Chum ,, | 6 | 0 |
| Kilchis River | Chum ,, | 2 | 0 |
| Kilchis River | Silver (Jacks) | 1 | 0 |
| Tenmile Lakes | Silver ,, | 40 | 0 |
| Tenmile Lakes | Silver (Adults) | 144 | 0 |
| Total | | 207 | 0 |
| Marked Fish Taken at Hatcheries | | | |
| Big Creek Hatchery | Silver (Adults) | 164 | 164 |
| Nehalem Hatchery | Silver ,, | 70* | 70* |
| Little Nestucca River | Silver (Jacks) | 1 | 1 |
| Total | | 235 | 235 |
| Unmarked Fish Taken at Hatcheries | | | |
| Klaskanine Hatchery | Silver (Jacks) | 86 | 28 |
| Klaskanine Hatchery | Silver (Adults) | 30 | 14 |
| Nehalem Hatchery | Silver ,, | 14 | 7 |
| South Coos Hatchery | Silver ,, | 10 | 9 |
| Total | | 140 | 58 |

* Includes 1 fish marked at the Nehalem Hatchery and recovered in Big Creek.

## NOCARDIAL DISEASES

It was recently shown that nocardial infections occur in several species of freshwater and marine fishes (Heuschmann-Brunner, 1965). Some of these diseases had mistakenly been attributed to mycobacteria, which is not surprising since *Nocardia* spp. are acid-fast and produce symptoms and gross pathology in fishes which is similar to that produced by mycobacteria. Studies with *Nocardia* isolated from neon tetra (Conroy, 1963a; Valdez and Conroy, 1963) and rainbow trout (Snieszko, Bullock, Dunbar and Pettijohn, 1964) indicated these organisms were *N. asteroides* (Gordon and Mihm, 1962). As with *Mycobacterium* spp., *Nocardia* grow in compact masses and produce swelling like that seen in the infected rainbow trout (Fig. 32). A stained smear from the affected area shows the masses of organisms present (Fig. 33). Experimental infection could not be established by feeding fingerling and adult rainbow trout pelleted food heavily seeded with the organism, and only an occasional trout could be infected by intraperitoneal injection of the nocardial cells. A lesion with *Nocardia* could not be demonstrated by examination of stained smears until one to three months after injection (Snieszko *et al.*, 1964). In the neon tetra, there was ulceration of

Figure 32. Infected rainbow trout (*Salmo gairdneri*) fingerlings with distended abdomen caused by growth of *Nocardia asteroides*. Scale is in millimeters. (Snieszko, Bullock, Dunbar, and Pettijohn, 1964)

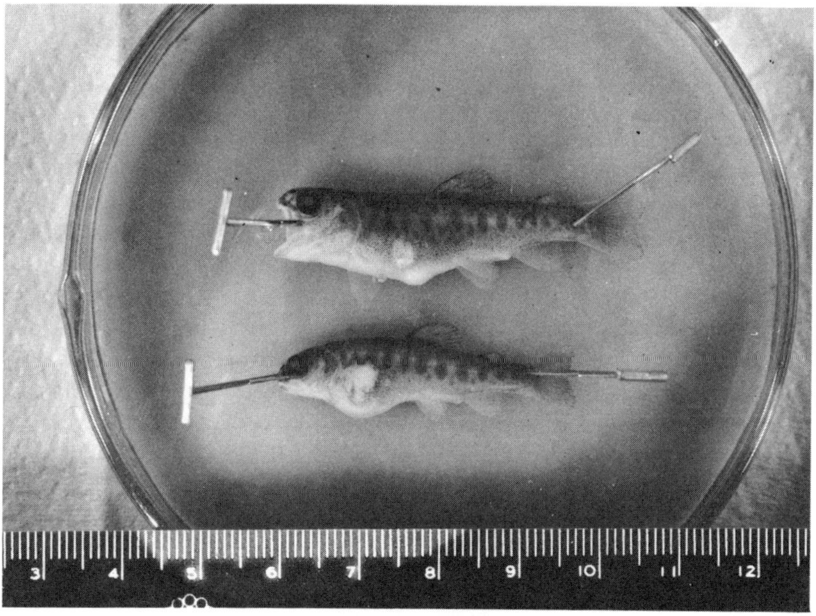

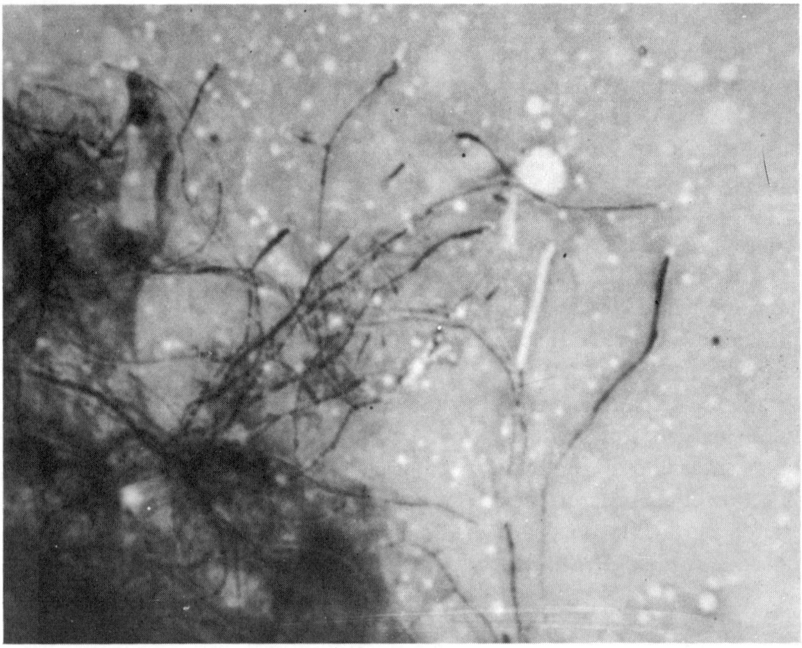

Figure 33. *Nocardia asteroides* stained directly from distended abdomen of infected fish. ×1500. (Snieszko, Bullock, Dunbar, and Pettijohn, 1964)

the body surface, listlessness, loss of appetite, and emaciation (Conroy and Valdez, 1962). Another nocardial infection in rainbow trout was recently reported in Germany (Heuschmann-Brunner, 1966). *N. asteroides* was also isolated from brook trout in aquaria. The kidneys of the brook trout were granular and the posterior one-third of the kidney in most trout was hard and rubbery. Some fish also had hemorrhagic gonads (Campbell and Mackelvie, 1968).

An infection caused by acid-fast bacilli was found in a rainbow trout kept three years in an aquarium. Emaciation, anemia, caseous kidneys, and testicular atrophy were the chief pathological changes. The organism could not be cultured and other bacteria were at times isolated. Rainbow trout injected intraperitoneally with infected, ground kidneys died in thirteen to fourteen days with exudative changes, whereas guinea pigs developed abscesses at the injection site. A chub (*Gila* sp.) was found to be refractory to infection. It was postulated that the infection was caused by a *Nocardia* alone or by a *Mycobacterium* together with other bacteria (Ghittino, 1966b).

## STREPTOMYCES

An organism similar to a *Nocardia* but not acid-fast was isolated from blueback salmon (Rucker, 1949). Though experimental infection could not be established by feeding the bacterium, intraperitoneal or intramuscular injection of the organism into salmon would produce mortality about a week after injection and thirty-seven of forty injected salmon died within sixty-four days after injection.

Intramuscular injection produced a necrotic lesion which spread slowly whereas intraperitoneal injection resulted in mycelial masses along the intestine (Fig. 34) and more diffuse growth on and in various tissues. Histological examination of an affected liver showed a mycelial mass on the surface and hyphae penetrating and causing an underlying focal necrosis (Fig. 35) but no significant inflammatory response.

Figure 34. Nodules of *S. salmonicida* on the viscera of an inoculated blueback salmon (*Oncorhynchus nerka*). ×1.5. (Rucker, 1949)

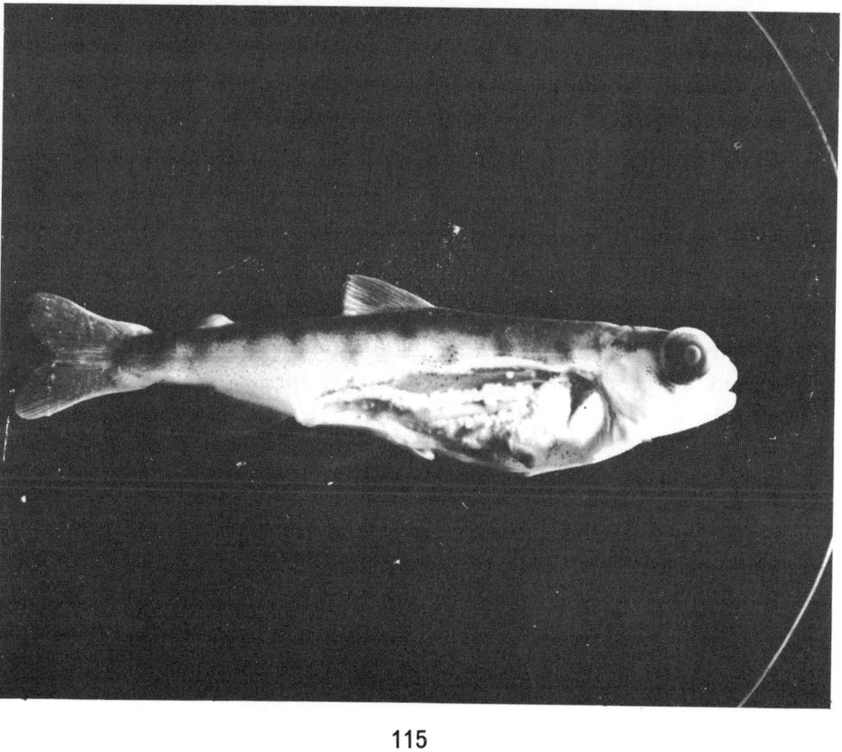

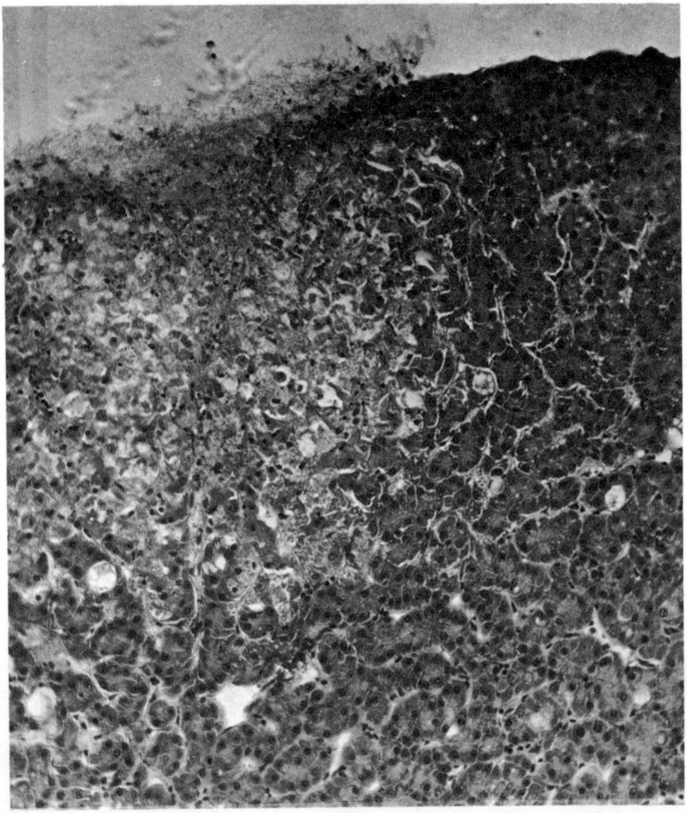

Figure 35. Liver of blueback salmon (*Oncorhynchus nerka*) fingerling with *S. salmonicida* on the surface at the left showing an underlying area of focal necrosis. Normal tissue is at the right. ×150. (Rucker, 1949)

A study of the characteristics of the isolate indicated that it should be placed in the genus *Streptomyces* and a new species *S. salmonicida* was proposed.

Another streptomycete disease apparently occurred in seahorses (*Hippocampus* sp.) (Mackie, *et al.*, 1935). When this organism was injected into three-spine sticklebacks (*Gasterosteus aculeatus*) it grew in compact masses which displaced normal tissue, but did not invade other tissue. The organism was classified as a *Streptothrix*.

# Less Common Bacterial Diseases

## Introduction

Fish diseases caused by bacteria described to this point are fairly accurately known, widely distributed, and occur with some degree of regularity. Diseases described below occur infrequently, or sporadically, and for this reason were studied less extensively. Their etiology may often be uncertain and methods of control were either insufficiently tested or unknown.

## DISEASES CAUSED BY FLAVOBACTERIA

### Definition of the Disease

Fish diseases caused by flavobacteria are defined as diseases in which infection with well-identified flavobacteria was established as their etiology.

### Historical

There have been several reports of flavobacteria causing disease in freshwater and marine fishes. A flavobacterium was isolated from heart blood of a dace and shown to be pathogenic to trout, roach, carp, gudgeon, and minnow (Brisou, Tysset and Vacher, 1959) and several flavobacterial species were isolated from diseased dace, gudgeon, and roach (Brisou *et al.*, 1959). A granulomatous disease among black mollies (*Mollienesia sphenops*) was attributed to a *Flavobacterium* sp. (Kluge, 1965) and produced experimental infection in this species.

Mortalities among marine fishes during periods of "red tide" have been attributed to an organism presently classified as *F. piscicida* (Bein, 1954). Studies have shown this bacterium produces a powerful neuromuscular toxin which kills several species of fishes.

### Symptoms and Pathology

Symptoms and pathology produced by flavobacteria resemble those produced by other gram-negative bacteria and have included hemorrhagic lesions in the musculature, swelling of the liver, splenomegaly, and hypertrophy of the gall bladder (Brisou *et al.*, 1959). The flavobacterial disease in black mollies was characterized by granulomas in internal organs, brain, and meninges. Exophthalmia was produced by granulomas in the optic nerve, orbit, and retina. *F. piscicida* produces a neuromuscular type of toxin which is absorbed from the water by fishes and causes aimless swimming, disturbance of equilibrium, spasms, convulsions, and finally paralysis and death (Meyer, Baslow, Bein, and Mark, 1959).

### Diagnosis

The isolation from diseased fish of a gram-negative, usually non-motile, rod-shaped bacterium producing a yellow to orange pigment is tentative diagnosis of flavobacteria-caused disease. Characteristics of the isolate would have to be examined in order to determine the species and whether it really belongs in the genus *Flavobacterium.*

### Etiology

Unlike ulcer disease or furunculosis, no well-defined single species of *Flavobacterium* causes all flavobacterial diseases of fishes. Flavobacteria are generally characterized as gram-negative, asporogenous rods which produce a yellow to orange, water-insoluble pigment. Most species are non-motile but some are motile by means of peritrichous flagella. One point should be clarified in regard to classification. French workers group motile strains as *Flavobacterium* but non-motile strains are classified in the genus *Empedobacter*. In contrast, American classification has both motile and non-motile forms as *Flavobacterium* sp. (Breed *et al.*, 1957). In this text the American classification will be followed. Among the species listed in the seventh edition of *Bergey's Manual* (Breed *et al.*, 1957), *F. balustinum* and *F. piscicida* have been reported as fish pathogens. *Flavobacterium vadosa* and *F. lacunatum* have also been reported as fish pathogens, but at present do not appear in *Bergey's Manual*. The *Flavobacterium* producing granulomatous lesion in black mollies was not speciated. Also recent investigations of *F. piscicida* have shown that this organism is polar flagellated and probably belongs in the genus *Pseudomonas* (Buck, Meyers and Leifson, 1963).

### Transmission, Pathogenesis, Host, and Geographic Range

Transmission of some flavobacterial diseases has probably been by means of external parasites in the sense that the parasites would create a portal of entry for the bacteria (Brisou *et al.*, 1959). Since flavobacteria occur in water, direct transmission from fish to fish is probable once a disease is established.

Pathogenesis may be accomplished by endotoxin in some species and by a powerful neuromuscular-type toxin by *F. piscicida.*

Presumably marine, freshwater, and aquarium species are susceptible to infrequent infection.

## DISEASES CAUSED BY PASTEURELLA

WHITE PERCH PASTEURELLOSIS

During the summer months of 1963 a massive kill of white perch (*Roccus americanus*), and to a lesser extent of striped bass (*R. saxatilis*), occurred on the east coast of the United States in the Chesapeake Bay and its inflowing streams. Localized, small, fish kills often occurred in this area, but this kill was very large, with losses of white perch in the millions. Many aspects of the epizootic are available and this kill presents interesting information

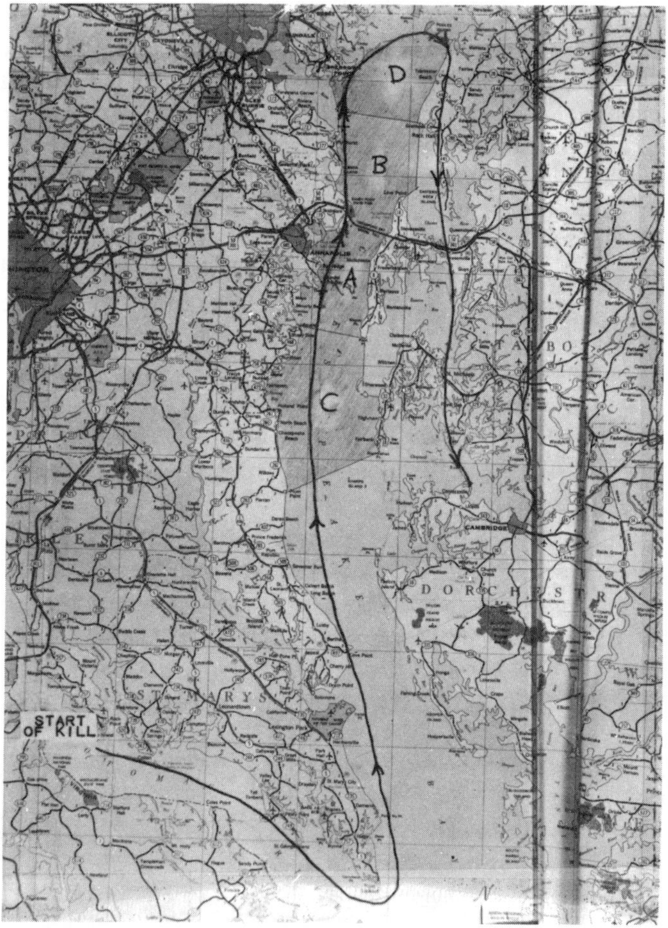


Figure 36. Disease course of the 1964 white perch (*Roccus americanus*) epizootic in Chesapeake Bay. Kill appeared to be most severe in shaded areas A, B, C, D.

on an infectious disease in the estuarine environment. Mortalities began in June in the lower Potomac River (Fig. 36) and it was first thought that this was another localized kill. However, the white perch continued to die in ever-increasing numbers and the affected area spread during July and August into the entire bay area and tributary rivers (Fig. 36). The shaded area in Fig. 36 indicates the area of heaviest kill. Many possible causes were given for the kill and included: 1. toxic algae bloom, 2. pollution, 3. toxic agent selective for white perch, 4. physical factors such as low level of dissolved oxygen. In July, preserved white perch collected in the area of original mortality in the Potomac River were sent to the Eastern Fish Disease Laboratory for examination. Microscopic examination of kidney tissue showed large numbers of gram-negative, polar-staining bacteria (Fig. 37) identified as a *Pasteurella* sp. (Snieszko, Bullock, Hollis, and Boone, 1964). Subsequently the same type of bacterium was found to occur in pure culture in moribund white perch from throughout the bay. The white perch population was quite high and organic pollution in the bay and rivers offered enrichment for algae and also bacteria. Although the source of the *Pasteurella* is not known, later studies indicated it was not part of the flora of normal white perch (Allen and Pelczar, 1967). Since the striped bass appeared to have a chronic infection, they may have been the source of the bacterium. The combination of physical and environmental stress, large white perch population with no prior exposure to the *Pasteurella* may have

Figure 37. The *Pasteurella* from white perch (*Roccus americanus*). Note the bipolar staining. ×1500.

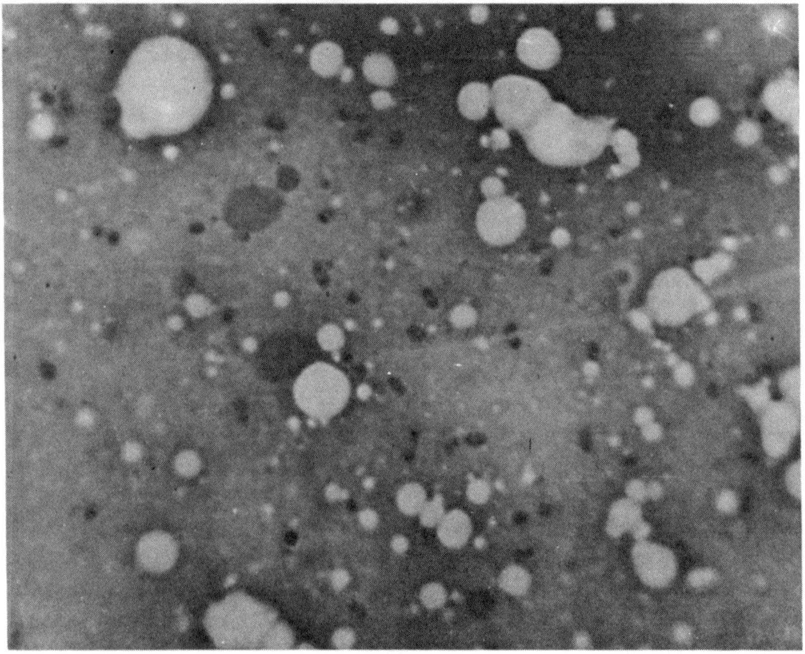

provided the necessary conditions for the explosive epizootic. Since no mortalities of white perch infected with the *Pasteurella* have since appeared, one might assume that the susceptible individuals have been killed or environmental conditions have improved, or perhaps both. The bacterium has been tentatively classified as *Pasteurella piscicida* (Janssen and Surgalla, 1968).

One important point to remember is that fish epizootics in the estuarine or marine environment probably follow the same pattern as the epizootic which occur in freshwater cultured fishes.

### OTHER PASTEURELLA FROM FISH

A *Pasteurella* species different in some characteristics from the white perch bacterium was isolated from diseased perch, chub, and rudd (*Scardinius erythrophthalmus*). Perch showed no gross pathology but rudd and chub showed skin lesions, hemorrhagic areas in the muscle, and congestion in kidney, liver, and spleen. The consistent isolation of the *Pasteurella* sp. and its presence in large numbers in liver and kidney of diseased fishes implicated the bacterium as the probable etiologic agent (Ajmal and Hobbs, 1967).

### DISEASES CAUSED BY STREPTOCOCCUS AND LACTOBACILLUS

What appears to be the first recorded instance of a streptococcal infection of fish has been described by Hoshina, Sano and Morimoto (1958). These workers isolated a species of *Streptococcus* from diseased rainbow trout in Japan during the months of March and April, 1957, and noted that the mortality rate was extremely high, reaching approximately 0.3% per day. The causative organism was isolated from the liver and kidney of a number of diseased fishes, and almost invariably was obtained in pure culture from these organs. It proved to be a gram-positive, non-motile, non-acid-fast, and non-encapsulated coccus, occurring in pairs or in short chains. The individual cells measured 0.62–0.65μ in diameter. On agar plates, it produced small whitish-colored colonies. This organism grew on plates of culture media containing bile salts, and was a facultative aerobe. Hoshina, *et al.* (1958) considered their isolate to belong to the non-hemolytic enterococci (Lancefield's Group D), and suggested that it was a strain of *Streptococcus faecalis* differing only in relation to optimum pH and temperature requirements, and to the source from which it had been isolated.

The diseased fish were generally normal in appearance, except in advanced cases when they became sluggish. On autopsy the anus and intestine showed symptoms of marked congestion, and the latter organ contained a small amount of reddish-tinged mucoid fluid. The kidney was notably swollen, although in all cases its coloration appeared normal. The liver was of a dark red color, and showed well-defined congestion. Microscopical examination of smears prepared from the liver, kidney, spleen, and heart blood showed the presence of cocci. The pathology of this disease gave a picture of disintegration and necrosis of the heart, kidney, and liver tissues. The principal organs affected were the intestines, in which severe destruction of the epithelial tissues was observed. The muscular tissue was inflamed, and the blood vessels of the sub-epithelial connective tissues were likewise markedly inflamed. Cellular infiltration was detected in the sub-epithelial and muscular tissues. Small zones of necrosis were observed in the liver. In the kidney the cavities of the renal tubules were filled with degenerative epithelial cells. Degenerative changes were also detected in the endocardial musculature of the heart. As these workers pointed out, the disease which they describe bears very little resemblance to other diseases of the salmonids, and more so in the complete absence of external lesions in the skin and musculature. In contrast, the infection is typified by enteritis, hepatitis, and enlargement of the kidney. Of special interest is the fact that the fish hatchery from which the diseased specimens were obtained was situated in very propitious surroundings, fresh spring water being led thereto by means of a concrete pipe directly from the source. This tends to discount any possibility of infiltration by sewage contaminated water. It was suggested therefore that the original source of infection might have been contaminated food.

More recently, a group β hemolytic *Streptococcus* sp. was isolated from two epizootics among golden shiners (*Notemigonus crysoleucas*). Diseased fish exhibited numerous raised, inflamed areas along the dorso-lateral regions of the body, with the area just anterior to the caudal peduncle most frequently attacked. Lesions erupted as the disease progressed. The disease was transmissible by adding a diseased fish to an aquarium containing healthy fish, and by exposing healthy fish to a suspension containing $10^7$ organisms per milliliter and then placing them into aquarium water. Disease could not be transmitted by adding the *Streptococcus* sp. directly to aquarium water. When injected intraperitoneally, the bacterium was lethal to bluegills, green sunfish (*Lepomis cyanellus*), and American toads (*Bufo americanus*), but not to goldfish, big mouth buffalo (*Ictiobus cyprinellus*), black crappie (*Pomoxis salmoides*), and channel catfish. Homoiothermic animals were not susceptible (Robinson and Meyer, 1966).

Only one instance of a disease in fish caused by lactobacilli appears to have been recorded in the literature. Rucker, Earp and Ordal (1954) described an infection of coho salmon as being caused by a species of *Lactobacillus*. The disease was characterized principally by the presence of large muscular abscesses, and although the course of the infection was slow and chronic, a large percentage of the fish was eventually lost.

#### DISEASES CAUSED BY MICROCOCCI (STAPHYLOCOCCI)

Anderson (1911) described a disease of plaice, haddock, and whiting, which he believed to have been caused by a staphylococcal infection. The symptoms included an ulcer which at times extended through the muscles to the vertebral column, and in places the skin had a wrinkled appearance, suggesting that the infection had extended beneath the integument. The eyes were frequently destroyed, and the bones of the head were attacked. Anderson suggested that the infection might have been brought about by sewage-borne bacteria. Egana (1945) briefly mentions a disease of gudgeon (*Gobio fluviatilis*) supposedly caused by "*Micrococcus pyogenes aureus*," but does not further elaborate.

A disease of rainbow trout in Argentina possibly caused by a micrococcus was described by Conroy (1966a). The disease became apparent in the mature adults in a private fish hatchery from San Carlos de Bariloche. The presence of circular lesions of a greyish-white color was observed on the dorsal surface of the fish, but without any obvious hemorrhage. Internally there was a slight inflammation of the anal region of the intestine, and a slight enlargement of the spleen. The other internal organs were apparently quite normal. The blood picture of the diseased fish did not differ markedly from the normal values for this species. A non-motile and gram-positive micrococcus was isolated from the heart blood of two fish, and shown to be sensitive to Streptomycin, Terramycin, Kanamycin, Chloromycetin, Aureomycin, and Rifomycin. It was not possible to carry out pathogenicity tests with rainbow trout, but this organism was shown to be non-pathogenic to goldfish following intra-peritoneal injection.

### DISEASES CAUSED BY BACILLUS AND BACTERIUM

(Except for the corynebacterial kidney disease described above, there are very few reports of fish diseases attributed to gram-positive rods.)

The vast majority of the bacterial fish pathogens described in the past as *Bacillus* or *Bacterium* are now recognized as belonging to other genera (e.g. *Bacillus anguillarum*, *Bacterium salmonicida*). However there exists a small number of diseases from which have been isolated organisms classified as belonging to one or the other of these two genera, and where the characteristics of the organisms given are insufficient to allow a more detailed classification. One such disease has been described by van Duijn (1938), and was characterized by a pronounced lepidorthosis of small tropical aquarium fishes. The symptoms were of slow development, and led to a marked protusion of the scales. Ecchymoses were frequently present on the skin of the ventral surface; the fins were generally inflamed, and the causative organism was isolated from the majority of the body organs. Van Duijn described this organism as *Bacterium lepidorthosae*, a small gram-negative rod which was actively motile. The number and distribution of the flagella was not determined, and therefore it is difficult to decide to which genus the organism might belong. *B. lepidorthosae* ferments lactose, fails to produce acetylmethylcarbinol, and gives a positive methyl red test. This suggests a certain similarity between the organism and members of the coli-aerogenes group, but the precise classification of the isolate must remain in doubt. It does not appear in the present edition of *Bergey's Manual* (Breed *et al.*, 1957).

Unless the skin had previously been damaged, healthy fish failed to develop symptoms following exposure to aquarium water known to contain the bacterium. Van Duijn observed that the most susceptible species are the Siamese fighting fish (*Betta splendens*), the paradise fish (*Macropodus opercularis*), and the cyprinodonts. Platys appeared to be more resistant.

Lepidorthosis can be treated effectively by addition of sulfanilamide at a rate of about 200 milligrams per liter, or chloramphenicol at a rate of 15 milligrams per liter of water in which the infected fishes are kept (van Duijn, 1967).

# Literature Cited

Ajmal, M., and B. Hobbs. 1967. Species of *Corynebacterium* and *Pasteurella* isolated from diseased salmon, trout and rudd. Nature 215: 142–143.

Alexander, D. M. 1913. A review of piscine tuberculosis with a description of an acid-fast bacillus found in the cod. Rept. Lancs. Sea-Fish Lab. 21: 42–49.

Allen, N., and M. Pelczar. 1967. Bacteriological studies on the white perch *Roccus americanus*. Chesapeake Sci. 8: 135–154.

Allison, L. 1957. Variation in strength of pyridylmercuric acetate technical and its effect on rainbow trout. Prog. Fish-Cult. 19: 108–111.

Allison, Leonard N. 1958. Multiple sulfa therapy of kidney disease among brook trout. Prog. Fish-Cult. 20 (2): 66–68.

Amend, D. F., J. L. Fryer, and S. K. Pilcher. 1965. Production trials utilizing sulfonamide drugs for the control of "coldwater disease" in juvenile coho salmon. Res. Briefs, Fish Comm. of Oregon 11 (1): 14–17.

Amlacher, E. 1956. Das Serum und Gallenbilirubin normaler und künstlich mit *Pseudomonas punctata forma ascitae* (Zimmermann) Schäperclaus infizierter Karpfen ($K_2$). Arch. Fischereiwiss. 7.

—— 1957. Der Blutzucker normaler und an Infektiöser Bauchwassersucht erkrankter Karpfen ($K_2$). Arch. Fischereiwiss. 8.

—— 1961. Taschenbuch der Fischrankheiten. Gustaf Fischer Verlag, Jena. 286 p.

Anche, E. Amlacher, and J. Hobbs. 1897. Action de la tuberculose more injectée dans la cavité peritoneale des grenouilles. Compt. rend. soc. Biol. 49: 929.

Anderson, A. G. 1911. Bacteriological investigations as to the cause of an outbreak of disease amongst the fish at the marine laboratory, Bay of Nigg, Aberdeen. 28th Ann. Rept., Fish Bd. Scotland. 1909, Part 3, Sci. Invest., 38 p.

Anderson, J. I. W., and D. A. Conroy. 1969(a). Vibrio disease in marine fishes. IN: Diseases of Fishes and Shellfishes. Symposium of the Amer. Fish. Soc. In press.*

———— 1969(b). The pathogenic myxobacteria with special reference to fish disease. Jour. Appl. Bacteriol. 32: 30–39.

Aronson, J. D. 1926. Spontaneous tuberculosis in saltwater fish. J. Infec. Dis. 39: 315–320.

Axelrod, H. R. 1962. Diseases of tropical fishes. TFH Publications Inc., Jersey City. 32 p.

Baage, J., and O. Baage. 1956. *Vibrio anguillarum* som arsag til ulcussydom hos torks (*Gadus callarias,* Linné). Nord. veterinaermed. 8: 481–492.

Babes, V., and P. Riegler. 1903. Über eine Fischepidemie bei Bukarest. Zentrabl. Bakteriol., Abt. 1, Orig. 23: 438.

Bailey, Reeve M. (chairman). 1960. A list of common and scientific names of fishes from the United States and Canada. Amer. Fish. Soc., Special Publication No. 2.

Baker, J. A., and W. A. Hagan. 1942. Tuberculosis of Mexican platyfish (*Platypoecilus maculatus*). J. Infec. Dis. 70: 248–252.

Bandt, H. J. 1959. Wassertrübungen und Fische. Deutsche Fischerei. Ztg. 11: 321–322.

*Published in 1970, Special Publication No. 5, pp. 266-272.

Bataillon, E., Dubard, and L. Terre. 1897. Un nouveau type de tuberculose. Compt. rend. soc. Biol. 49: 446–449.

—— and L. Terre. 1897. La forme saprophytique de la tuberculose humaine et de la tuberculose aviaire. Compt. rend. soc. Biol. 124: 1399.

—— A. Moeller, and L. Terre. 1902. Über die Identität des Bacillus des Karpfens (Bataillon, Dubard, and Terre) und des Bacillus der Blindschleiche (Moeller). Z. Tuberk. 3: 467–468.

Bauer, O. N., and A. V. Uspenskaya. 1959. (Novye lechebnye sredstva bor'by s zabolevaniyami ryb). Proc. Conf. on Fish diseases, 19–25. (Trans from Russian, OTS 61–31058).

Bein, S. J. 1954. A study of certain chromogenic bacteria isolated from "Red Tide" water with a description of a new species. Bull. Mar. Sci Gulf and Caribbean. 4: 110–119.

Belding, David L., and B. Merrill. 1935. A preliminary report upon a hatchery disease of the Salmonidae. Trans. Amer. Fish. Soc. 65: 76–84.

Bell, G. 1961. Two epidemics of apparent kidney disease in cultured pink salmon. (*Oncorhynchus gorbuscha*) J. Fish Res. Bd. Can. 18: 559–562.

Bergman, A. 1909. Die rote Beulenkrankheit des Aals. Ber. Kgl. Bayer. Biolog. Versuch. München. 2: 10–54.

Bertarelli, E., and J. Bocchia. 1910. Neue Untersuchungen über Tuberkulose der Kaltblütter. Zentrabl. Bakteriol. Abt. 1. Orig. 54: 385–393.

Besse, P. 1949 Epizootie à bacilles ácido-résistentes chez de poissons exotiques. Bull. Acad. Vét. France. 23: 151–154.

Bojalil, L. F., J. Cerbón, and A. Trujillo. 1962. Adansonian classification of mycobacteria. J. Gen. Microbiol. 28(2): 333–346.

Borg, A. 1948. Studies on myxobacteria associated with diseases in salmonid fishes. Thesis. Univ. Washington, Seattle. 162 p.

—— 1960. Studies on myxobacteria associated with diseases in salmonid fishes. Wildlife Dis. 8: 1–85 (2 microcards).

Bott, T., J. Deffner, E. McCoy, and E. M. Foster. 1964. *Clostridium botulinum* type E. in fish from the Great Lakes. J. Bact. 91: 919–924.

Bottomley, P. E. and D. G. Holland. 1966. Columnaris disease in coarse fish. Assoc. of River Authorities Year Book, Westminster, London, S.W.1. England. 101–109.

Braude, A. 1964. Bacterial endotoxins. Sci. Amer. 210 (3): 36–45.

Breed, R. S., E. G. D. Murray, and N. R. Smith. 1957. Bergey's manual of determinative bacteriology. Seventh Edition, Williams and Wilkins Co., Baltimore, 1094 p.

Brisou, J., C. Tysset, and B. Vacher. 1959. Recherches sur les Pseudomonadaceae. Études de deux souches de *Flavobacterium* isolées des poissons d'eau douce. Ann. Inst. Pasteur. 96: 633.

Brunner, G. and R. Striegel-Jaxtheimer. 1951. Die Bakteriellen Erreger der infecktiösen. Bauchwassersucht der Karpfen. Allg. Fischerei-Ztg. 76 (19): 393.

———— 1953. Pseudomonas granulata (nov. spec.) Zooparasiten und fischpathogene Keime im Abwasser und Fischwasser. Münchner Beiträge zur Abwasser, – Fischerei- und Flussbiologie, R. Oldenbourg, Munchen, Heft I: 109–119.

Bryant, M. Jr. 1951. The use of PMA in treating columnaris. Prog. Fish-Cult. 13: 103–104.

Buck, J. D., S. P. Meyers, and E. Leifson. 1963. *Pseudomonas (Flavobacterium) piscicida* Bein Comb. nov. J. Bacteriol. 86: 1125–1126.

Bückmann, A. 1952. Infektionen mit *Glugea stephani* und mit Vibrio anguillarum bei Schollen (*Pleuranectes platessa* L.) Kurze Mitt. Fisch. Max-Plank-Inst. Meersebiol. 1: 1–7.

Bullock, G. L. 1965(a). Simple enrichment of commercial media for growth of *Hemophilus piscium*. Prog. Fish-Cult. 27: 163–164.

—— 1965(b). Characteristics and pathogenicity of a capsulated *Pseudomonas* isolated from goldfish. Appl. Microbiol. 13: 89–92.

—— 1966. Precipitin and agglutinin reactions of aeromonads isolated from fish and other sources. Bull. Off. Int. Epizoot. 65 (5–6): 805–824.

—— 1968. The bacteriology of brook trout with tail rot. Prog. Fish-Cult. 30(1): 19–22.

—— 1970. Studies on selected fish pathogenic mycobacteria and bacterial gill disease in hatchery-reared salmonids. Thesis, Fordham Univ., N.Y., 121 p.

——and D. W. McDaniel. 1968. Effect of temperature on immunized goldfish and rainbow trout. IN: Progress in Sport Fishery Research for 1967. Bur. Sp. Fish. and Wildl., Resource Publ. 64, p. 20.

—— S. F. Snieszko, and C. E. Dunbar. 1965. Characteristics and Identification of oxidative pseudomonads isolated from diseased fish. J. Gen. Microbiol. 38: 1–7.

Burrows, R. 1964. Effect of accumulated excretory products on hatchery-reared salmonids. U.S. Fish. Wildl. Serv., Bur. Sp. Fish. Wildl., Research Report 66. 12 pp.

—— and D. Palmer. 1949. Pyridlmercuric Acetate: its toxicity to fish, efficacy in disease control, and applicability to a simplified treatment technique. Prog. Fish-Cult. 11 (3): 147–151.

Busing, K. H. 1952. *Pseudomonas hirudinis*, ein bakterieller Darmsymbiont des blutegels (*Hirudo officinalis*). Zentrabl. Bakteriol. Parasitenk. Infektionsk. Hyg., I orig. 157: 478–484.

Calkins, G. 1899. Report upon the recent epidemic among brook trout (*Salvelinus fontinalis*) on Long Island, N.Y. Comm. Fish, Game, and Forests, Ann. Rept. 4 (1898): 175–189.

Campbell, G., and R. M. Mackelvie. 1968. Infection of brook trout (*Salvelinus fontinalis*) by Nocardiae. J. Fish. Res. Bd. Can. 25: 423–425.

Caselitz, Fredrich-Hermann. 1966. Pseudomonas-Aeromonas und ihre humanmedizinische Bedeutung. Ver. Gustav Fisher. Verlag Jena, XII plus 243 p.

Chaussinand, R., and P. Besse. 1951. Inoculation de bacille de Hansen et du bacille de Stefansky à la perche arc-en-ciel. Rev. Brasil. Leprol. 19: 4–7.

Chiesa, J. A. L. 1945. Enfermedades de los peces y criterio sanitario a observarse en las mismas. IN: "Peces" Talleres Gráficos Ferrari and Saccone, Buenos Aires. p. 228.

Chodyniecki, A. 1964. Wplyw kilkakrotnych iniekcji detreomycyny na stan zdrowotny kroczków karpia. Acta Hydrobiol. 6 (2): 87–96.

—— 1965. Serologiczne badania porównawcze antygenów somatyczmych szczepów *Aeromonas punctata* Zimmermann wyosobnionych w przebiegu posocznicy karpi. Acta Hydrobiol. 7 (2–3): 269–278.

Christensen, N. O., M. Jensen, and C. J. Rasmussen. 1963. Fish diseases in Denmark. Bull. Off. Int. Épiz. 50 (1/2): 21–29.

Clark, H. Fred, and Charles C. Shepard. 1963. Effect of environmental temperature on infection with *Mycobacterium marinum* (Balnei) of mice and a number of porkilothermic species. J. Bacteriol. 86 (5): 1057–1069.

Clement, Mary T., and N. E. Gibbons. 1960. *Aeromonas hydrophila (Pseudomonas hydrophila)* NRC 491 and NRC 492 established as *Aerobacter cloacae*. Can. J. Microbiol. 6 (5): 591–593.

Colgrove, D. J., and J. W. Wood. 1966. Occurrence and control of *Chondrococcus columnaris* as related to Fraser River sockeye salmon. Int. Pacific Salmon Fish Comm., Progress Report No. 15, 51 p.

Connell, F. 1937. Chlorine treatment for bacterial fin rot of trout. Prog. Fish-Cult. No. 34: 6–9.

Conroy, D. 1961(a). La producción de la putrefacción de la aleta caudal en los peces por la acción de *Aeromonas punctata*. Microbiol. Españ. 14: 233–238.

—— 1961(b). Las causas de un brote de putrefaccion de la aleta caudal en los peces y su tratamiento con kanamicina. Microbiol. Españ. 14: 239–246.

—— 1962. El tratamiento de "Tail rot" en peces con la Kanamicina. Ciencia e invest. 18: 133.
—— 1963(a). Otras observaciones sobre la putrfección de la aleta caudal en los peces. Microbiol. Españ. 16: 63–66.
—— 1963(b). Studies on the application of Kanamycin to the control and treatment of some bacterial fish diseases. J. Appl. Bacteriol. 26: 82–192.
—— 1963(c). The study of a tuberculosis-like disease in neon tetras (*Hyphessobrycon innesi*) I. Symptoms of the disease and preliminary description of the organism isolated. Microbiol. Españ. 16: 47.
—— 1964. Tail rot in fish. Nature (London). 201: 732–733.
—— 1965. Observaciones sobre casos espontaneos de la tuberculosis pisciaría. Microbiol. Espan. 18.
—— 1966(a). A report on the problem of bacterial fish diseases in the Argentine Republic. Bull. Off. Int. Epiz. 65 (5–6): 755–768.
—— 1966(b). Observaciones sobre casos espontáneos de tuberculosis íctica. Microbiol. Españ. 19: 93–113.
—— and E. B. Solarolo. 1965. Sensitivity of some acid-fast bacteria of piscine origin to certain chemotherapeutic substances. J. Fish. Res. Bd. Can. 22:243–245.
—— and I. E. Valdéz. 1962. Un caso de tuberculosis en peces tropicales. Rev. Latinoamer. Mircobiol. 5: 9–16.
—— and I. E. Valdéz. 1964. Una contribución al estudio de la tuberculosis pisciaria. Gac. Veterinaria. Bs. As., 26: 6p.
Cruz, J. da Costa. 1938. "Mycobacterium fortuitum," um novo bacilo acido-resistente patogenico para o homem. Acta Medica. Apr. 298–301.
David, H. 1927. Uber eine durch Choleraänliche Vibrionen hervorgerufene Fischseuche. Zentrabl. Bakteriol., Abt. 1, Orig. 102: 46–60.
Davis, G. W. G., and R. W. A. Park. 1962. A taxonomic study of certain bacteria currently classified a *Vibrio* species. J. Gen. Microbiol. 27: 101–119.
Davis, H. S. 1922. A new bacterial disease of fresh-water fishes. Bull. Bur. Fish. XXXVIII, Doc. 924: 261.
—— 1926. A new gill disease of trout. Trans. Amer. Fish Soc. 56: 156–160.
—— 1946. Care and disease of trout. Revised edition. U.S. Fish Wildl. Ser., Research Report No. 12. 98 p.
—— 1953. Culture and diseases of game fishes. Univ. Calif. Press, Berkeley. 332 p.
Deufel, Josef. 1967. Vorbeugende Behandlung der Furunkulose in der Forellenzucht mit Zinkbacitracin. Allg. Fischerei Ztg. 92 Jahrgang, Nr. 4.
Dombrowski, H. 1953(a). Bakterium oder Virus? Eine Stellungnahme zur Frage des Erregers der Infektiösen Bauchwassersucht des Karpfens. Fischwirt. Nr. 3.
—— 1953(b). Die Nahrungsmenge des Fischegels *Piscicola geometra L.* Biol. Zentralbl. 72: 311–314.
—— 1953(c). Untersuchungen über das Blut des Karpfens (*Cyprinus carpio* L.) und einiger anderer Süsswasserfischarten. Biol. Zentralbl. 72 Bd. Heft 3/4, 182–195.
Drouin de Bouville, R. 1907. Les maladies des poissons d'eau douce d'Europe Ann. Sci. Agron., 1: 120–250.
Duff, D. 1932. Investigators summary: Elk River investigation. Biol. Bd. Can. Ann. Rep. 1931. p. 71.
—— 1942. The oral immunization of trout against *Bacterium salmonicida*. J. Immunol. 44: 87–94.
van Duijn, C. 1938. Beitrag zur Kenntnis der Schuppensträubung bei Fischen. Woch. Aquar. Terrar. 35: 68.
—— 1967. Diseases of fishes. Sec. Ed. Iliffe Books Ltd. London. 309 p.
Dworkin, M. 1966. Biology of the Myxobacteria. Ann. Rev. Microbiol. 20: 75–106.
Dyk, V. 1953. Vice péče vodám ohroženým furunkulosou. Ceskoslov Rybárstvi 3: 40–41.

Earp, B. J., C. H. Ellis, and E. J. Ordal. 1953. Kidney disease in young salmon. Special Report Series No. 1. State of Wash. Dept. of Fisheries.

Eddy, B. P. 1960. Cephalotrichous, fermentative gram-negative bacteria, the genus *Aeromonas*. J. Appl. Bacteriol. 23 (2): 216–249.

—— 1962. Further studies on *Aeromonas*. I. Additional strains and supplementary biochemical tests. J. Appl. Bacteriol. 25 (2): 137–146.

Ehlinger, N. F. 1964. Selective breeding of trout for resistance to furunculosis. N.Y. Fish Game J. 11 (2): 78–90.

Eicher, C. 1947. Dual treatment for bacterial fin rot. Prog. Fish-Cult. 9: 94–95.

Embody, G., and C. Hayford. 1925. The advantage of rearing brook trout fingerlings from selected breeders. Trans. Amer. Fish. Soc. 55: 135–148.

Emmerich, R., and C. Weibl. 1894. Üeber eine durch Bakterien erzeugte Seuche unter den Forellen. Arch. Hyg. Bakteriol. 21: 1–21.

Ewing, W., R. Hugh, and J. G. Johnson. 1961. Studies on the *Aeromonas* group. Pub. Health Serv. Comm. Disease Center, Atlanta. 37 p.

Field, J. B., L. L. Gee, C. A. Elvehjem, and C. Juday. 1944. The blood picture in furunculosis induced by *Bacterium salmonicida* in fish. Arch. Biochem. 3: 277–284.

Fijan, N. 1968. The survival of *Chondrococcus columnaris* in waters of different quality. Bull. Off. Int. Épiz. 69 (7–8): 1159–1166.

—— L. J. Kunst, and I. Tomasěc. 1967. O. Liječenju zarazne vodene bolesti šarana nekim antibioticima i furazolidonom. Vet. Arh. (Zagreb). 37 (1–2): 34:45.

Fish, F. 1934. Ulcer disease of trout. Trans. Amer. Fish. Soc. 64: 252–258.

—— 1937. Furunculosis in wild trout. Copeia, 37–40.

—— 1947. Disease control in hatchery fish. U.S. Fish Wildl. Ser., Fishery Leaflet 222. 10 p.

—— and Robert R. Rucker. 1945. Columnaris as a disease of cold-water fishes. Trans. Amer. Fish. Soc. 73 (1943): 32–40.

Flemming, H. 1958. Untersuchungen über die Bluteiwesskörper gesunder und bauchwassersuchtskranker Karpfen. Z. Fischerei. N.F. 7: 91–152.

Foster, R., and P. Olsen. 1951. An incident of high mortality among large rainbow trout after treatment with pyridylmercuric acetate. Prog. Fish-Cult. 13: 129–130.

Garnjobst, Laura. 1945. *Cytophaga columnaris* (Davis) in pure culture: A myxobacterium pathogenic to fish. J. Bacteriol. 49: 113–128.

Gee, L., and W. Sarles. 1942. The disinfection of trout eggs contaminated with *Bacterium salmonicida*. J. Bacteriol. 44: 111–126.

Ghittino, P. 1963. Les maladies des poissons en Italie. Bull. Off. Int. Épiz. 50. (1/2): 59–87.

—— 1966(a). Suggestions pour l'établissement di une Liste internationale des Maladies Contangieuses des Poissons. Bull. Off. Int. Épiz. 65: 1165–1172.

—— 1966 (b). Observations sur l'infection par bactéries acido-alcoolo-résistantes chez la truite arc-en-ciel. Bull. Off. Int. Épiz. 65: 772–792.

—— 1967. Eziologia e lesioni anatomo-patologiche della Malattia Branchiale (MB) delle trotelline in Italia. Rev. It. Piscic. Ittiopat. A. 11 N. 2 24–29.

Gibbs, Erich L. 1963. An effective treatment for red-leg disease in *Rana pipiens*. Lab. Animal Care. 13 (6): 781–783.

Gilardi, Gerald. 1967. Morphological and biochemical characteristics of *Aeromonas punctata* (*hydrophila, liquefaciens*) isolated from human sources. Appl. Microbiol. 15 (2): 417–421.

Glantz, P. J., and G. E. Krantz. 1965. *Escherichia coli* serotypes isolated from fish and their einvironment. Health Lab. Sci. 2: 54–63.

Goncharov, G. D. 1959. Virusnaya krasnukha ryb v SSSR i za rubezhom. (Virus dropsy of fish in the USSR and abroad). Trudy Soveshchanii, Ikhtiol. Komissiya Akad. Nauk SSSR. 9: 34–38.

——1965. Rubella, a viral fish disease. IN: Viral Diseases of Poikilothermic Vertebrates. Ann. N.Y. Acad. Sci. 126 (Art 1): 598–600.

Gordon, Ruth E., and Joan Mihm. 1962. The type species of the genus *Nocardia*. J. Gen. Microbiol. 27 (1): 1–10.
Gräf, W. 1963(a). Die zytopathogen Eigenschaften der anaeroben Myxobakterien. Arch. Hyg. Bakteriol. 146: 481–491.
—— 1963(b). Die pathogenitat anaerober Myxobakterien (Sphaerocytophaga) in Tierversuch. Arch. Hyg. Bakteriol. 146: 492–500.
Grassl, E. F. 1957. Possible value of continuous feeding of medicated dry diets to prevent and control pathogens in hatchery-reared trout. Prog. Fish-Cult. 19 (2): 85–88.
von Gravenitz, A., and A. H. Mensch. 1968. The genus *Aeromonas* in human bacteriology. N. Engl. J. Med. 278: 245–249.
Griffin, P. J. 1951. Cocarboxylase and adenosine triphosphate as growth factors for *Hemophilus piscium*. Arch. Biochem. 30(1): 100–102.
—— S. F. Snieszko, and S. B. Friddle. 1953(a). A more comprehensive description of *Bacterium salmonicida*. Trans. Amer. Fish. Soc. 82: 129–138.
—— 1953(b). Pigment formation by *Bacterium salmonicida*. J. Bacteriol. 65: 652–659.
—— 1953(c). A new adjuvant in the diagnosis of fish furunculosis caused by *Bacterium salmonicida*. Vet. Med. 48: 280–282.
Gutsell, James. 1946. Sulfa drugs and the treatment of furunculosis in trout. Science 104: 85–86.
—— 1948. The value of certain drugs especially sulfa drugs in the treatment of furunculosis in brook trout, *Salvelinus fontinalis*. Trans. Amer. Fish. Soc. 75: 186–199.
—— and S. F. Snieszko. 1949(a). Response of brook, rainbow and brown trout to various dosages of sulfamerazine. Trans. Amer. Fish. Soc. 77: 93–101.
—— 1949(b). Dosage of sulfamerazine in the treatment of furunculosis in brook trout (*Salvelinus fontinalis*). Trans. Amer. Fish. Soc. 76 (1946): 82–96.
Haley, Richard, Sterling P. Davis, and Jackson M. Hyde. 1967. Environmental stress and *Aeromonas liquefaciens* in American and threadfin shad mortalities. Prog. Fish-Cult. 27 (4): 193.
Halvelka, J., and F. Volf. 1965. Dalši poznatky o používání antibiotik v našem rybářství. Bul VUR Vodnany 1 (3): 12–20.
Halver, J. 1954. Fish diseases and nutrition. Trans. Amer. Fish. Soc. 83: 254–261.
Hayashi, K., S. Kobayashi, T. Kamata, and H. Ozaki. 1964(a). Studies on the vibrio disease of rainbow trout (*Salmo gairdneri irideus*). I. Therapeutic effect of the nitrofuran derivatives. J. Fac. Fish., Prefect. Univ. Mie. 6: 171–180.
—— 1964(b). Studies on the vibrio disease of rainbow trout (*Salmo gairdneri irideus*). II. Prophylactic vaccination against the vibrio disease. J. Fac. Fish., Prefect. Univ. Mie. 6: 181–191.
Herman, Roger Lee. 1968. Fish furunculosis 1952–1966. Trans. Amer. Fish. Soc. 97 (3): 221–230.
Herr, E. 1901. Ein Beitrag zum Verhalten der Tuberkelbazillen bei überimpfung auf Blindschleichen. Hyg. Infektion., 38: 198.
Heuschmann, Otto. 1952. Bauchwassersucht bei Regenbogenforellen? Allg. Fischerei-Ztg. 77 (11): 214–215.
—— 1953. Teichversuche zur Frage der Bekämpfungsmöglichkeit der ansteckenden Bauchwassersucht des Karpfens. Zooparasiten und fischpathogene Keime im Abwasser und Fischwasser. Münchner Beitr. Abwasser-Fisch Flussbiol, Heft I: 76–108.
Heuschmann-Brunner, G. 1965. Nocardiose bei Fischen des Süsswassers und des Meeres. Tierarztl. Wochensch. 78 Jahrgang. Heft 5: 94–95.
—— 1966. Nocardia Infektion bei Regenbogen forellen (*Salmo gairdneri*). Tierärtzl. Wochensch. 79 Jahrgang. Heft 5: 96–97.
Hewetson, A. 1962. Furunculosis in salmon kelts. Nature (London) 194: 312.
Hewitt, E. R. 1937. Fin rot eliminated by continued tank sterilization. Prog. Fish-Cult. No. 33: 19–20.

Hodgkiss, W., and J. M. Shewan. 1950. Pseudomonas infection in a plaice. J. Pathol. Bacteriol. LXII (4): 655–657.

Hofer, Bruno. 1904. Handbuch der Fischkrankheiten. München, Verlag des Allg. Fischerei-Ztg., 359 p.

Hoshina, Toshikazu. 1956. An epidemic disease affecting rainbow trout in Japan. J. Tokyo Univ. of Fisheries. 42 (1): 15–16.

—— 1962. On a new bacterium, *Paracolobactrum anguillimortiferum* n. sp. Bull. Jap. Soc. Sci. Fish. 28: 1.

—— Tokuo Sano, and Yoshimasa Morimoto. 1958. A streptococcus pathogenic to fish. J. Tokyo Univ. Fish. 44: 57–68.

Hunn, J. B. 1964. Some patho-physiologic effects of kidney disease in brook trout. Proc. Soc. Exp. Biol. Med. 117: 383–385.

Irwin, W. 1959. Terramycin as a control for fin rot in fishes. Prog. Fish-Cult. 21 (2): 89–90.

Isom, Billy G. 1960. Outbreaks of columnaris in Center Hill and Old Hickory Reservoirs, Tennessee. Prog. Fish-Cult. 22 (1): 43–45.

Ivlev, V. S. 1955. The effect of winter conditions on the blood of some freshwater fishes. (In Russian). Biull. Moskovskovo Obschchestva Ispytatelei Prirody. Biol. 60 (4): 73–78. (Biol. Abstr. 31 (7): 20,000, 1957).

Jahnel, J. 1940. Spontaninfektion mit saurefesten Stabchen bei Fischen. Neue Beobachtungen uber Fischtuberkulose. Wein. Tierarztl. Monatsschr. 27: 289.

Janssen, W. A., and M. T. Surgalla. 1968. Morphology, physiology, and serology of a *Pasteurella* species, pathogenic for white perch (*Roccus americanus*). J. Bacteriol. 96: 1606–1610.

Johnson, Harlan E., and Richard F. Brice. 1953. Mortality of silver salmon from treatments with sulfamerazine. Prog. Fish-Cult. 15 (1): 31–32.

Johnstone, J. 1913. Diseased conditions of fishes. Rept. Lancs. Sea-Fish. Lab. 21: 20–25.

Kabaivanski, Ja., H. Slavkov, D. Savov, and St. Stanoe. 1954. Crevna forma nov furunkuloza po pstrvite u nas. Izvestija Mikrobiol. Inst. Blg. Akad. na naukite 5: 267–275.

Karlsson, K. A. 1964. Serologische studien von *Aeromonas salmonicida*. Zentralbl. Bakteriol. 1 Orig. 194: 73–80.

Kingsbury, O. R. 1961. A possible control of furunculosis. Prog. Fish-Cult. 23 (3): 136–137.

Klingler, K. 1958. Entzündliche Kiemenschwellung bei Regenbogenforellen. Schweiz. Fischerei-Ztg. 66: 98–99.

Klontz, G. W. 1966. Immunopathology. IN: Progress in Sport Fishery Research, 1965, Bur. Sp. Fish. and Wildl. Resource Publ. 17: 11–12.

—— W. T. Yasutake and A. J. Ross. 1966. Bacterial diseases of the Salmonidae in the Western United States: Pathogenesis of furunculosis in rainbow trout. Amer. J. Vet. Res. 27 (120): 1455–1460.

Kluge, John P. 1965. A granulomatous disease of fish produced by Flavobacteria. Pathol. Vet. 2: 545–552.

Kocylowski, B. 1963. État actuel des maladies des poissons. Organisation de l'inspection des poissons et de leurs produits de consommation en Pologne. Bull. Off. Int. Épiz. 50 (1/2): 89–109.

Krantz, G. E., J. M. Reddecliff, and C. E. Heist. 1963. Development of antibodies against *Aeromonas salmonicida* in trout. J. Immunol. 91 (6): 757–760.

—— 1964. Immune response of trout to *Aeromonas salmonicida*. Part II. Evaluation of feeding techniques. Prog. Fish-Cult. 26: 65–69.

Kubota, S. S., and K. Hagita. 1963. Studies on the diseases of marine culture fishes. II. Pharmaco-dynamic effects of nitrofurazone for fish diseases (I). J. Fac. Fish., Prefect. Univ. Mie 6: 125–144.

—— —— Kakakuwa. 1963. Studies on the diseases of marine-culture fishes. I. General description and preliminary discussion of fish diseases at the Mie Prefecture. J. Fac. Fish. Univ. Mie., 6: 107–124.

Lennon, Robert E. and Phillip S. Parker. 1960. An outbreak of columnaris disease in stonerollers. Prog. Fish-Cult. 22 (3): 102.

Lewis, William M. and Michael Bender. 1960. Heavy mortality of golden shiners during harvest due to a bacterium of the genus *Aeromonas*. Prog. Fish-Cult. 22 (1): 11–14.

—— 1961. Free-living ability of a warm-water fish pathogen of the genus *Aeromonas* and factors contributing to its infection of the golden shiner. Prog. Fish-Cult. 23 (3): 124–126.

Li, M. F., and Carol Flemming. 1967. A proteolytic pseudomonad from skin lesions of rainbow trout (*Salmo gairdneri*). I. Characteristics of the pathogenic effects and the extracellular proteinase. Can. J. Microbiol. 13: 405–416.

Liebmann, H. 1963. The study of diseases of fish and the organization of their control in Western Germany. Bull. Off. Int. Épiz. 50 (1/2): 5–20.

—— K. Offhaus and S. Riedmuller. 1960. Electrophoretische Blutuntersuchunger bei normalen und bauchwassersuchtkranken Karpfen. Allg. Fischerei Ztg. 85: 502–505.

Liu, P. V. 1961. Observations on the specificities of extracellular antigens of the genera *Aeromonas* and *Serratia*. J. Gen. Microbiol. 24: 145–153.

Ljajman, E. 1949. Kurs bolezney ryb. Food Industry Publications. Moscow. 306 p. (In Russian).

Ljunberg, O. 1963. Report on fish diseases and inspection of fish products in Sweden. Bull. Off. Int. Épiz. 50 (1/2): 111–120.

Lubarsch, O. 1900. Über das Verhalten der Tuberkelpilze in Froschkörpren. Zentralbl. Bakteriol., Abt. 1, Orig. 28: 421.

Lucky, Z. and J. Vanek. 1962. Tuberkuloza u Akvarijnich ryb. Sb. Vys. Sk. Zemed. V Brne X (XXXI): 127–131.

—— E. Mesaros, and V. Pleva. 1962. Prispevek k. etiologii infekcni vodnatelnosti kapru. Sb. Vy. Sk. Zemed. V. Brne X (XXXI): 113–122.

Machado-Cruz, J. 1962. Sur l'apparition récente de "bacterial gill disease" en Europe et sa caracterisation histopathologique. Instituto de Zoologia "Dr Augusto Nobre", Faculdade de Ciencias do Porto 82: 18 p.

Mackie, T. J., J. A. Arkwright, T. E. Pryce-Tannatt, J. C. Mottram, W. D. Johnston, and W. J. M. Menzies. 1930. Furunculosis Committee Report. Interim. H.M. Stationery Office, Edinburgh. 65 p.

—— 1933. Second interim report of the Furunculosis Committee. H.M. Stationery Office, Edinburgh. 81 p.

—— 1935. Furunculosis Committee Report. Final. H.M. Stationery Office, Edinburgh. 67 p.

Maestrone, G. and M. A. Benjaminson. 1962. Leptospira infection in the goldfish (*Carassius auratus*). Nature (London) 195: 719–720.

Manion, R., S. Bradley, H. Zinneman, and W. Hall. 1964. Interrelationships among mycobacteria and nocardiae. J. Bacteriol. 87: 1056–1059.

Margolis, L. 1954. Ulcer disease and furunculosis in a Quebec trout hatchery. Can. Fish Cult. No. 15, 2 p.

Marsh, M. 1902. *Bacterium truttae*, a new species of bacterium pathogenic to trout. Science N.S. 16 (409): 706–707.

—— 1905. The Cold Spring Harbor epidemic among trout. N.Y. Forest, Fish and Game Comm. Ann. Rept. 10: 125–139.

Mattheis, T. 1966. Zur Desinfektion von Teichböden. Z. Fischerei 14 (5/6): 337–346.

Matthey, R. 1963. Rapport sur les maladies des poissons en Suisse. Bull. Off. Int. Épiz. 50 (1/2): 121–126.

McCraw, B. M. 1952. Furunculosis of fish. U.S. Fish and Wildl. Serv., Spec. Sci. Rep. Fish. 84. 87 p.

Meyer, Fred P. 1964. Field treatments of *Aeromonas liquefaciens* infections in golden shiners. Prog. Fish-Cult. 26 (1): 33–35.

—— and J. D. Collar. 1964. Description and treatment of a *Pseudomonas* infection in white catfish. Appl. Microbiol. 12 (3): 201–203.

Meyers, S. P., M. H. Baslow, S. J. Bein, and C. E. Marks. 1959. Studies of *Flavobacterium piscicida* Bein. I. Growth, toxicity, and ecological considerations. J. Bacteriol. 78: 225.

Michelson, Edward. 1961. An acid-fast pathogen of freshwater snails. Amer. J. Trop. Med. Hyg. 10 (3): 423–433.

Nicolas, J., and C. Lesieur. 1899. Effects de l'ingestion des crachats tuberculeaux humaine chez les poissons. Compt. Rend. Soc. Biol. 51: 774.

Nigrelli, Ross F. 1943. Causes of diseases and death of fishes in captivity. Zoologica 28 (22): 203–216.

—— 1953. Two diseases of the neon tetra, *Hyphessobrycon innessi*. Aquarium J. 24: 203–308.

—— and S. H. Hutner. 1945. The presence of a myxobacterium, *Chondrococcus columnaris* (Davis) Ordal and Rucker (1944), on *Fundulus heteroclitus* (Linn). Zoologica 30 (2): 101–105.

—— and Henry Vogel. 1963. Spontaneous tuberculosis in fishes and in other cold-blooded vertebrates with special reference to *Mycobacterium fortuitum* Cruz from fish and human lesions. Zoologica 48 (9): 130–143.

—— S. Jakowski, and H. Baker. 1957. A bacterial disease of cichlids in captivity. Aquarium 26 (7): 233–235.

Nowotny, A. 1969. Molecular aspects of endotoxic reactions. Bacteriol. Rev. 33 (1): 72–98.

Nybelin, O. 1935. Untersuchengen uber deu bei Fischen Krankheitserregenden spaltpilz *Vibrio anguillarum*. Medd. undersokn-Anst. Sotvattensfisk. Stockh: No. 8, 62 p.

Ojala, O. 1963. Fish diseases in Finland. Bull. Off. Int. Épiz. 50 (1/2); 31–42.

Oppenheimer, C. 1958. A bacterium causing tail rot in Norwegian codfish. Inst. Mar. Sci. 5: 160–162.

—— 1963. On marine fish diseases. IN: Fish as Food, 2. Academic Press Ltd., London and New York.

Ordal, E. J., and B. J. Earp. 1956. Cultivation and transmission of etiological agent of kidney disease in salmonid fishes. Proc. Soc. Exp. Biol. Med. 92: 85–88.

—— and R. R. Rucker. 1944. Pathogenic myxobacteria. Proc. Soc. Exp. Biol. Med. 56: 15–18.

Otte, Elmar. 1963. Die heutigen Ansichten über die Ätiologie der Infektiösen Bauchwassersucht der Karpfen. Wien. Tierärztl. Monatsschr. 50 (11): 995–1005.

Pacha, R. 1968. Characteristics of *Cytophaga psychrophila* (Borg) isolated during outbreaks of bacterial coldwater disease. Appl. Microbiol. 16: 97–101.

—— and E. J. Ordal, 1963. Epidemiology of columnaris disease in salmon. Bacteriol, Proc., p. 3.

Page, L. A. 1961. Experimental ulcerative stomatitis in king snakes. Cornell Vet. LI: 258 266.

Parisot, Thomas J. 1958. Tuberculosis of fish. Bacteriol. Rev. 22: 240–245.

—— and A. Decker. 1960. A comparative study of the causative agent of a mycobacterial disease of salmonid fishes. I. A comparison of the staining characteristics of the fish disease with human tuberculosis in sections stained by Fite-Faraco and Ziehl-Neelson methods. Amer. Rev. Resp. Dis. 81: 60–67.

—— and James W. Wood. 1966. Fish mycobacteriosis (tuberculosis). U.S. Bur. Sp. Fish. and Wildl., FDL-7.

Pentelow, F. 1947. Freshwater fish. IN: UFAW Handbook on The Care and Management of Laboratory Animals. Ballière Tindall and Cox Ltd., London. 263 p.

Piper, Robert G. 1961. Toxic effects of erythromycin thiocyanate on rainbow trout. Prog. Fish-Cult. 23 (3): 134–135.

Plehn, M. 1924. Praktikum der Fischkrankheiten. E. Schweizerbartische Verlagsbuchhandlung, Stuttgart. 301-479.

Post, G. 1959. A preliminary report on the use of nitrofuran compounds for furunculosis of trout, with special emphasis on furoxone. Prog. Fish-Cult. 21 (1): 30–33.

—— 1963. The immune response of rainbow trout (*Salmo gairdneri*) to *Aeromonas hydrophila*. Utah Dept. Fish and Game, Dept. Information Bull. 63–7.

—— 1965. A review of advances in the study of diseases of fish: 1954–64. Prog. Fish-Cult. 27 (1): 3–12.

—— and R. E. Keiss. 1962. Further laboratory studies on the use of furazolidone for the control of furunculosis of trout. Prog. Fish-Cult. 62 (1): 16–21.

Poston, H. 1966. Toxicity of the chemical form of vitamin A for trout. IN: Progress in Sport Fishery Research, 1965, Bur. Sp. Fish. Wildl. Resource Publ. 17: 17–18.

Rabb, L. and L. A. McDermott. 1961. Bacterial diseases of Ontario freshwater fish. Wildl. Dis., no. 19. (Micro-card).

Reddecliff, J. M. 1960. Immune response of trout to *Aeromonas salmonicida*. M.Sc. Thesis, Penn. State Univ. 107 p.

Reed, G. B., and G. C. Toner. 1941. Red sore disease of pike. Can. J. Res. 19 (5): 139–143.

Reichenbach-Klinke, H. 1966. Krankheiten und Schädigungen der Fische. Gustav Fischer Verlag, Stuttgart. 389 p.

Riddell, W., and D. Alexander. 1912. Note on an ulcerative disease of the plaice. Trans. Liverpool Biol. Soc. 26: 155–161.

Riedmüller, S. 1965. Elektrophoretische Bluteiweissuntersuchungen bei gesunden und kraken Karpfen. Allg. Fischerei Ztg. 18: 28–35.

Robinson, J., and F. Meyer. 1966. Streptococcal fish pathogen. J. Bacteriol. 92: 512.

Rock, Leo, and Harold M. Nelson. 1965. Channel catfish and gizzard shad mortality caused by *Aeromonas liquefaciens*. Prog. Fish-Cult. 27 (3): 138–141.

Roegner-Aust, S. 1953. Zur frage einer Virusätiologie bei verschiedenen Fischkrankheiten. Münchner Beitr. Abwasser-Fisch. Flussbiol. Heft 1: 120–145.

—— G. Brunner, and R. Jaxtheimer. 1950. Elektronenmikroskopische Untersuchungen über den Erreger der Infektiösen Bauchwassersucht der Karpfen—Bacterium?—Virus? Allg. Fischerei-Ztg. 75: 420–422.

Rogers, E., B. Hazen, S. Friddle, and S. F. Snieszko. 1951. The toxicity of pyridylmercuric acetate technical (PMA) to rainbow trout (*Salmo gairdneri*). Prog. Fish-Cult. 13: 71–73.

Rosner, Richard. 1964. *Aeromonas hydrophila* as the etiologic agent in a case of severe gastroenteritis. Amer. J. Clin. Pathol. 42: 402–404.

Ross, A. John. 1960. *Mycobacterium salmoniphilum* sp. nov. from salmonid fishes. Amer. Rev. Resp. Dis. 81 (2): 241–250.

—— 1963. Mycobacteria in adult salmonid fishes returning to national fish hatcheries in Washington, Oregon and California in 1958–59. U.S. Fish Wildl. Ser. Spec. Sci. Rept. Fish. No. 462.

—— and F. Brancato. 1959. *Mycobacterium fortuitum* Cruz from the tropical fish *Hyphessobrycon innesi*. J. Bacteriol. 78: 392–395.

—— and H. Johnson. 1962. Studies of transmission of mycobacterial infections in chinook salmon. Prog. Fish-Cult. 24 (4): 147–149.

—— and G. W. Klontz. 1965. Oral immunization of rainbow trout (*Salmo gairdneri*) against an etiologic agent of "red mouth disease." J. Fish. Res. Bd. Can. 22 (3): 713–719.

—— B. J. Earp, and J. W. Wood. 1959. Mycobacterial infections in adult salmon and steelhead trout returning to the Columbia River basin and other areas in 1957. U.S. Fish Wildl. Ser. Spec. Sci. Rept. Fish. No. 332.

—— J. E. Martin, and V. Bressler. 1968. *Vibrio anguillarum* from an epizootic in rainbow trout (*Salmo gairdneri*) in the U.S.A. Bull. Off. Int. Épiz. 69 (7–8): 1139–1148.
—— R. R. Rucker, and W. H. Ewing. 1966. Description of a bacterium associated with redmouth disease of rainbow trout (*Salmo gairdneri*). Can. J. Microbiol. 12: 763–770.
—— Phyllis Nordstrom, Jack E. Bailey, and John R. Heaton. 1960. A bacterial disease of yellow perch (*Perca flavescens*). Trans. Amer. Fish. Soc. 89 (3): 310–312.
Rucker, R. R. 1948. New compounds for the control of bacterial gill disease. Prog. Fish-Cult. 10 (1): 19–22.
—— 1949. A streptomycete pathogenic to fish. J. Bacteriol. 58 (5): 659–664.
—— 1959. Vibrio infections among marine and freshwater fishes. Prog. Fish-Cult. 21 (1): 22–25.
—— 1966. Redmouth disease of rainbow trout (*Salmo gairdneri*). Bull. Off. Int. Epiz. 65 (5–6): 825–830.
—— B. Earp, and R. Burrows. 1956. Lignasan for bacterial gill disease. Prog. Fish-Cult. 18 (2): 75–77.
—— B. Earp, and E. J. Ordal. 1954. Infectious diseases of Pacific salmon. Trans. Amer. Fish. Soc. 83: 297–312.
—— H. Johnson, and G. Kaydas. 1952. An interim report on gill disease. Prog. Fish-Cult. 14 (1): 10–14.
—— H. Johnson, and E. Ordal. 1949. An investigation of the bactericidal action and fish toxicity of two homologous series of quaternary compounds. J. Bacteriol. 57: 225–234.
—— A. F. Bernier, W. J. Whipple, and R. Burrows. 1951. Sulfadiazine for kidney disease. Prog. Fish-Cult. 13 (3): 135–137.
Rychlicki, Z., and St. Zarnecki. 1957. Die Zatorer Karpfenaufzuchtmethode und deren Einfluss auf die Beseitigung der Bauchwassersucht. Zeit. Fischerei 5, N.F. 5/6: 423–442.
Sanz Egaña, C. 1945. Enfermedades infecciosas de los peces. IN: La inspección veterinaria. Rev. Vet. Espana, Barcelona, p. 383.
Sato, S. 1962. Mycobacteria and fish. Repura 12: 27.
—— 1963. Niacin-producing ability of some mycobacteria, in particular of fish origin, with special reference to the relationships between these strains and atypical mycobacteria. 3rd Ann. Session American College of Physicians, Far East Region, Yokosuka, Japan. May.
Schäperclaus, W. 1926. Bacterium fluorescens—infektion und Geschwülstbildungen bei Aalen mit Versuchlucktem Angelhaken. Z. Fischerei 24. p. 157.
—— 1927. Die Rotseuche des Aales im Bezirk von Rugen und Stralsund. Z. Fischerei. 25: 99–128.
—— 1928. Die Hechtpest in Brandenburg und Rügen. Z. Fischerei 26. 343–366.
—— 1930. *Pseudomonas punctata* als Krankheitserreger bei Fischen, Untersuchungen über Susswasseraalrotseuche, Leibeshölenwassersucht der Cypriniden, insbesondere des Karpfens und Fleckenseuche der Weissfische. Z. Fischerei. 28: 289–370.
—— 1934. Untersuchungen über die Aalseuchen in deutschen Binnen- und Küstenwässern 1930–1933. Z. Fischerei. 32. 191–217.
—— 1939. Untersuchungen über die Ansteckende Bauchwassersucht des Karpfens und ihre Bekämpfung. Z. Fischerei. 37: 1–5, 6–99, 127–182.
—— 1954. Fischkrankheiten. Akademie Verlag, Berlin. 708 p.
—— 1956. Bekämpfung der infektiösen Bauchwassersucht der Karpfens durch Antibiotika. Z. Fischerei. 5 (1–2): 3–59.
—— 1958. Bewährung des Chloronitrins in der Teichwirtschaftlichen Praxis und neue Versuche über die Anwendbarkeit weiterer Breitspektrum-Antibiotica bei der Bekämpfung der infektiösen Bauchwassersucht des Karpfens. Z. Fischerei. 7 N.F.: 599–628.

—— 1959. Grossversuche mit Streptomycin zur Bekämpfung der infektiösen Bauchwassersucht des Karpfens. Deut. Fisch. Ztg. 6. 176–179.

—— 1965. Etiology of infectious carp dropsy. IN: Viral Diseases of Poikilothermic Vertebrates. Ann. N.Y. Acad. Sci. 126 (Art. 1): 587–597.

—— 1967. Probleme der Karpfenimmunität gegenüber *Aeromonas punctata* und Fragen der antigenen struktur des Bakteriums. Z. Fischerei. 15 N.F. (1–2): 129–138.

—— and M. Brauer. 1964. Bedeutung der Fluoreszenten für die Entstehung und Bekämpfung der infektiösen Bauchwassersucht der Karpfen. Z. Fischerei. 12: 75–96.

—— and H. Mann. 1939. I. Untersuchungen über die ansteckende Bauchwassersucht des Karpfens und ihre Bekämpfung I–V. Z. Fischerei. 37 (1): 137–182.

Seaman, Wayne R. 1951. Notes on a bacterial disease of rainbow trout in a Colorado hatchery. Prog. Fish-Cult. 13 (3): 139–141.

Shafer, W. B., and C. L. Davis. 1961. A bacteriologic and histologic study of skin granuloma due to *Mycobacterium balnei*. Amer. Rev. Resp. Dis. 84: 837.

Shechmeister, I., L. Watson, V. Cole, and L. Jackson. 1962. The effect of X-radiation on goldfish. I. The effect of X-radiation on survival and susceptibility of the goldfish *Carassius auratus* to infection by *Aeromonas salmonicida* and *Gyrodactylus* spp. Radiat. Res. 16: 89–97.

Shewan, J. M., G. Hobbs, and W. Hodgkiss. 1960(a). A determinative scheme for the identification of certain genera of gram-negative bacteria, with special reference to the pseudomonadaceae. J. Appl. Bacteriol. 23 (3): 379–390.

—— 1960(b). The pseudomonas and achromobacter groups of bacteria in the spoilage of marine white fish. J. Appl. Bacteriol. 23 (3): 463–468.

—— W. Hodgkiss, and J. Liston. 1954. A method for the rapid identification of certain non-pathogenic asporogenous bacilli. Nature (London) 173: 208–209.

Sindermann, C. 1966. Diseases of marine fishes. Advan. Mar. Biol. 4: 1–89.

—— 1970 *Principal Diseases of Marine Fish and Shellfish*; 369 pp., Academic Pr.

—— and A. Rosenfield. 1954. Diseases of fishes of the Western North Atlantic. I. Diseases of the sea herring (*Clupea harengus*). Maine Dept. Sea and Shore Fish., Res. Bull. 18. 23 p.

Sion, V. 1900. Der Einfluss des Organismus Kaltblutiger Tiere auf den Bacillus der menschlichen Tuberkulose. Zbl. Bakt., Abt. 1, Orig. 27: 710.

Smith, H. W. 1950. Chloromycetin in the treatment of red leg. Science 112: 274–275.

Smith, I. W. 1961. A disease of finnock due to *Vibrio anguillarum*. J. Gen. Microbiol. 24: 247–252.

—— 1962. Furunculosis in kelts. Dept. Agr. Fish. Scot., Freshwater and Salmon Fisheries Res. No. 27. 1–12.

—— 1963. The classification of "*Bacterium salmonicida*." J. Gen. Microbiol. 33 (2): 263–274.

—— 1964. The occurrence and pathology of Dee disease. Freshwater and Salmon Fisheries Res. 34: 1–12.

Smith, W. W. 1942. Action of alkaline acriflavine solution on *Bacterium salmonicida* and trout eggs. Proc. Soc. Exp. Biol. Med. 51: 324–326.

Snieszko, S. F. 1949. Pyridylmercuric acetate technical: its use in control of gill disease and some external parasitic infections. Prog. Fish-Cult. 11 (3): 153–155.

—— 1952. Ulcer disease in brook trout (*Salvelinus fontinalis*): Its economic importance, diagnosis, treatment and prevention. Prog. Fish-Cult. 14 (2): 43–49.

—— 1953. The disinfection of eyed trout eggs. Prog. Fish-Cult. 15 (1): 10.

—— 1958. Natural resistance and susceptibility to infections. Prog. Fish-Cult. 20 (3): 133–136.

—— 1959. Antibiotics in fish diseases and fish nutrition. Antibiot. Chemother. 9 (9): 541–545.

—— 1964. Remarks on some facets of epizootiology of bacterial fish diseases. Develop. Ind. Microbiol. 5: 97–100.

—— and S. B. Friddle. 1948. Disinfection of rainbow trout eggs with sulfomerthiolate. Prog. Fish-Cult. 10 (3): 143–149.

—— and S. B. Friddle. 1949. Prophylaxis of furunculosis in brook trout (*Salvelinus fontinalis*) by oral immunization and sulfamerazine. Prog. Fish-Cult. 11 (3): 161–168.

—— 1950. A contribution to the etiology of ulcer disease of trout. Trans. Amer. Fish. Soc. 78: 56–63.

—— 1951. Tissue levels of various sulfonamides in trout. Trans. Amer. Fish. Soc. 80 (1950): 240–250.

—— 1952. Further studies on factors determining tissue levels of sulfamerazine in trout. Trans. Amer. Fish. Soc. 81 (1951): 101–110.

—— and P. J. Griffin. 1955. Kidney disease in brook trout and its treatment. Prog. Fish-Cult. 17 (1): 3–13.

—— and G. L. Hoffman. 1963. Control of fish diseases. Lab. Animal Care 13 (3): 197–206.

—— and E. Wood. 1955. The effect of some sulfonamides on the growth of brook trout, brown trout and rainbow trout. Trans. Amer. Fish Soc. 84: 86–92.

—— C. E. Dunbar, and G. L. Bullock. 1959. Resistance to ulcer disease and furunculosis in Eastern brook trout, *Salvelinus fontinalis*. Prog. Fish-Cult. 21 (3): 111–116.

—— P. J. Griffin, and S. B. Friddle. 1950. A new bacterium (*Hemophilus piscium* n. sp.) from ulcer disease of trout. J. Bacteriol. 59: 699–710.

———— 1952. Antibiotic treatment of ulcer disease and furunculosis in trout. Trans. N. Amer. Wildl. Conf. 17: 197–213.

—— J. S. Gutsell, and S. B. Friddle. 1950. Various sulfonamide treatments of furunculosis in brook trout, *Salvelinus fontinalis*. Trans. Amer. Fish. Soc. 78 (1948): 181–188.

—— G. L. Bullock, C. E. Dunbar, and L. L. Pettijohn. 1964. Nocardial infection in hatchery-reared fingerling rainbow trout (*Salmo gairdneri*). J. Bact. 88 (6): 1809–1810.

—— G. L. Bullock, Edgar Hollis, and J. G. Boone. 1964. *Pasteurella* sp. from an epizootic of white perch (*Roccus americanus*) in Chesapeake Bay tidewater areas. J. Bacteriol. 88: 1814–1815.

—— W. Piotrowska, B. Kocylowski, and K. Marek. 1938. Badania bakteriologiczne i serologiczne nad bakteriami posocznicy karpi. Rozpray biologiczne z zakresu medycyny weterynaryjnej rolnictwa i hodowli 16 (1–2): 15 p.

Solacroup, J. 1963. Les maladies de poissons en France-Importance sanitaire et économique. Traitement. Bull. Off. Int. Epiz. 50 (1/2): 51–58.

Sorvatchev, K. F. 1957. Changes in proteins of carp blood serum during hibernation. Biochemistry (Biokhimiya) 22 (5): 822–827.

Spence, K. D., J. L. Fryer, and K. S. Pilcher. 1965. Active and passive immunization of certain salmonid fishes against *Aeromonas salmonicida*. Can. J. Microbiol. 11: 397–405.

Spiczakow, T. 1933. Posocznica karpi (Septicaemia haemorrhagica cyprinorum). Przeglad Rybacki VI. 253–265.

Steffens, W. 1964. Die Überwinterung des Karpfens (*Cyprinus carpio*) als physiologisches problem. Z. Fischerei. 12: 97–153.

Swift, S., and H. Cohen. 1962. Granulomas of the skin to *Mycobacterium balnei* after abrasions from a fish tank. N. Engl. J. Med. 267: 1244–1246.

Terre, L. 1902. Essai sur la tuberculose des vértébrés à sang froid. Étude de pathologie experimentale et comparée. Zbl. Bakt. Abt. 1, Orig. 33: 210.

Thaxter, R. 1892. On the *Myxobacteriaceae*, a new order of *Schizomycetes*. Bot. Gaz. 17: 389–406.

Tomašec, I. I., and N. N. Fijan. 1965. The etiology of infectious dropsy of carp. IN: Viral Diseases of Poikilothermic Vertebrates. Ann. N.Y. Acad. Sci. 126 (Art. 1): 606–615.
Toole, M., and W. Tiller. 1964. Minnow propagation: its problems and commercial possibilities. Texas Fish and Game Comm.
Tunison, A., and C. McCay. 1937. The nutrition of trout. Courtland Hatchery Report No. 6. N.Y. State Cons. Dept., Albany. 24 p.
Valdéz, I., and D. Conroy. 1963. The study of a tuberculosis-like condition in neon tetras (*Hyphessobrycon innesi*). II. Characteristics of the bacterium isolated. Microbiol Españ. 16: 249–253.
Valtis, J. 1932. Le virus tuberculeux. Masson et Cie. Paris. p. 58.
Van Horn, M., and M. Katz. 1946. Pyridylmercuric acetate as a prophylactic in fisheries management. Science 104: 557.
Vogel, H. 1958. Mycobacteria from cold-blooded animals. Amer. Rev. Resp. Dis. 77: 823.
Wagner, E. D. and Curtis Perkins. 1952. *Pseudomonas hydrophila,* the cause of "red mouth" disease in rainbow trout. Prog. Fish-Cult. 14 (3): 127–128.
Wakabayashi, Hisatsugn, and Synzo Egusa. 1967. Columnaris disease of the Japanese loach. Fish. Pathol. 1 (2): 20–26.
Wang, L., R. R. Colwell, T. E. Lovelace and G. E. Krantz. 1969. Isolation of *Vibrio parahaemolyticus* from Chesapeake Bay. Bact. Proceed. p. 1.
Warren, J. 1963(a). Kidney disease of salmonid fishes and the analysis of hatchery waters. Prog. Fish-Cult. 25 (3): 121–131.
—— 1963(b). Toxicity tests of erythromycin thiocyanate in rainbow trout. Prog. Fish-Cult. 25 (2): 88–92.
Wells, Nelson, and Claude E. Zobell. 1934. *Achromobacter ichthyodermis,* n. sp. the etiological agent of an infectious dermatitus of certain marine fishes. Proc. Natl. Acad. Sci. 20: 123–126.
Wolf, K. E. 1956. Survey on the occurrence of kidney disease in trout hatcheries in some inland states. Mimeo, Microb. Lab. U.S. Fish Wildl. Serv. 11 p.
—— 1966. The fish viruses. IN: Advances in Virus Research. 12: 35–101. Academic Press, Inc., New York.
——and C. E. Dunbar. 1959. Test of 34 therapeutic agents for control of kidney disease in trout. Trans. Amer. Fish Soc. 88: 117–124.
Wolf, L. E. 1937. An air bladder disease of lake trout fingerlings. Trans. Amer. Fish. Soc. 66: 359–363.
—— 1939. Observations on ulcer disease of trout. Trans. Amer. Fish. Soc. 68: 136–151.
—— 1941. Further observations on ulcer disease of trout. Trans. Amer. Fish. Soc. 70: 369–381.
—— 1947. Sulfamerazine in the treatment of trout for furunculosis and ulcer disease. Prog. Fish-Cult. 9 (3): 115–124.
—— 1954. Development of disease-resistant strains of fish. Trans. Amer. Fish Soc. 83 (1953): 342–349.
Wolter, R. 1960. Die *Vibrio-anguillarum*—Seuche im Strelsund und Greifswalder Bodden, Z. Fischerei. 9: 765–769.
Wood, E. M., and W. T. Yasutake. 1956(a). Histopathology of fish. III. Peduncle (cold-water) disease. Prog. Fish-Cult. 18 (1): 58–61.
—— 1956(b). Histopathology of fish. IV. A granuloma of brook trout. Prog. Fish-Cult. 18 (3): 108–112.
—— 1956(c). Histopathology of kidney disease in fish. Am. J. Pathol. XXXII (4): 845–857.
—— 1957. Histopathology of fish. V. Gill disease. Prog. Fish-Cult. 19 (1): 7–13.
—— and H. E. Johnson. 1957. Acute sulfamethazine toxicity in young salmon. Prog. Fish-Cult. 19 (2): 64–67.
—— and S. F. Snieszko. 1955. Sulfonamide toxicity in brook trout. Trans. Amer. Fish Soc. 84: 155–160.

Wood, J. W. 1959. Ichthyophthiriasis and furunculosis in adult pacific salmon. Prog. Fish-Cult. 21 (4): 171.

—— 1968. Diseases of Pacific salmon. Their prevention and treatment. Dept. Fish., Hatchery Div. State of Washington.

—— and Erling J. Ordal. 1958. Tuberculosis in Pacific salmon and steelhead trout. Fish Comm. of Oregon. Contribution no. 25: 38 p.

—— and J. Wallis. 1955. Kidney disease in adult chinook salmon and its transmission by feeding to young chinook salmon. Research Briefs, Fish. Comm. of Oregon. 6 (2): 32–40.

ZoBell, C. E., and N. A. Wells. 1934. An infectious dermatitis of certain marine fishes. J. Infec. Dis. 55: 299–305.

## INDEX

(References set in **boldface** indicate illustrations.)

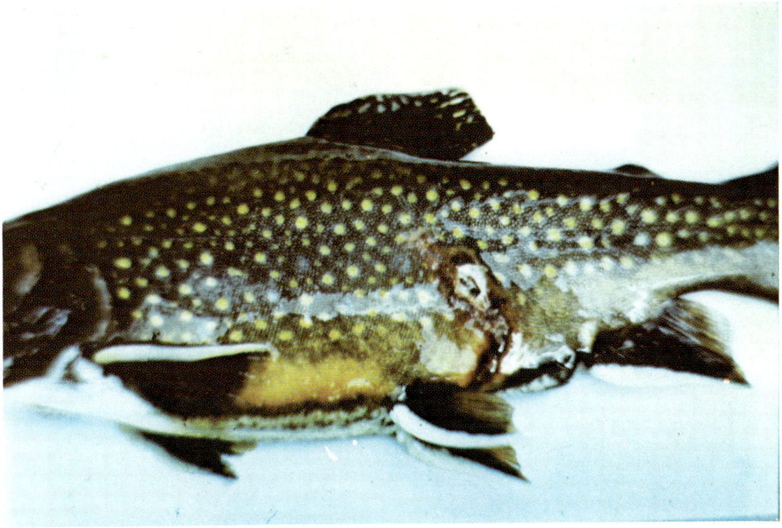

Figure 2. Adult brook trout (*Salvelinus fontinalis*) showing necrotic lesion from chronic furunculosis.

(See page 12)

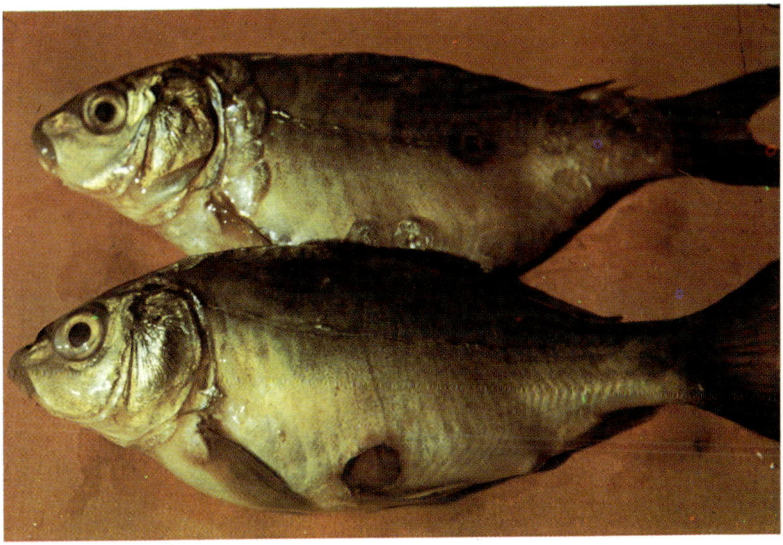

Figure 5. Carp (*Cyprinus carpio*) with ulcerative form of hemorrhagic septicemia. (Courtesy of Dr. Pietro Ghittino.)

(See page 23)

(See page 44)

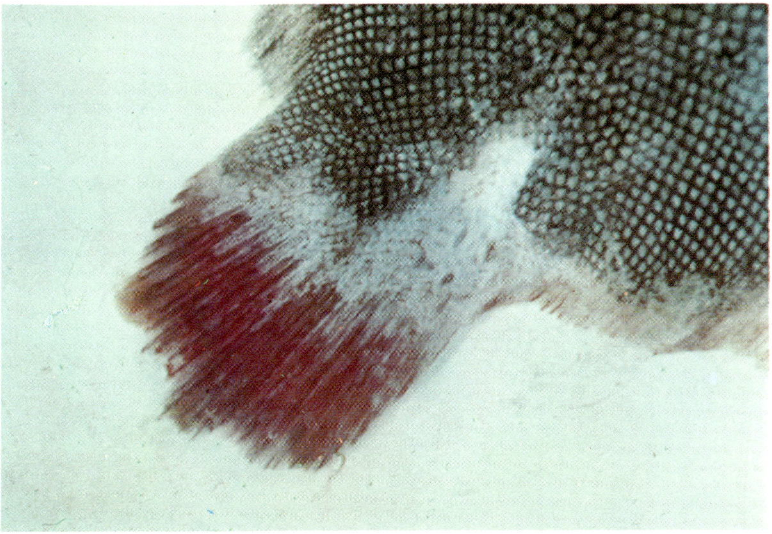

Figure 8. External pathology in Pleuronectidae caused by vibrio infections.
a. Tail rot in Dover sole (*Solea vulgaris*)
b. External lesions in lemon sole (*Pleuronectes microcephalus*).
(Courtesy of Dr. Iain Anderson)

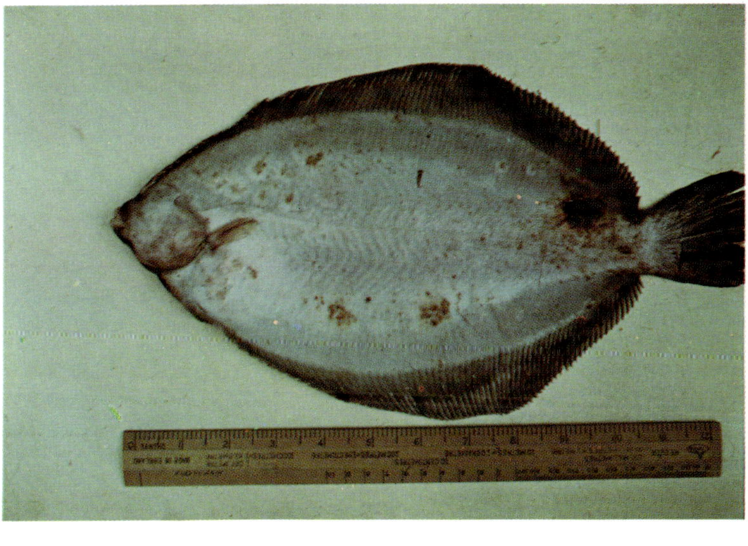

(See page 95)

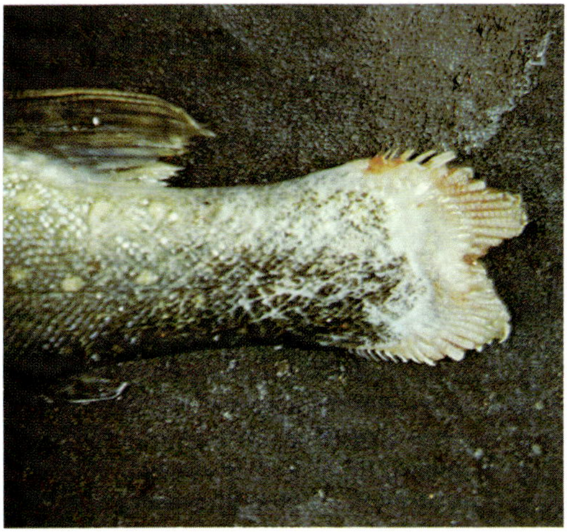

Figure 17. Advanced coldwater disease in brook trout (*Salvelinus fontinalis*) yearling.

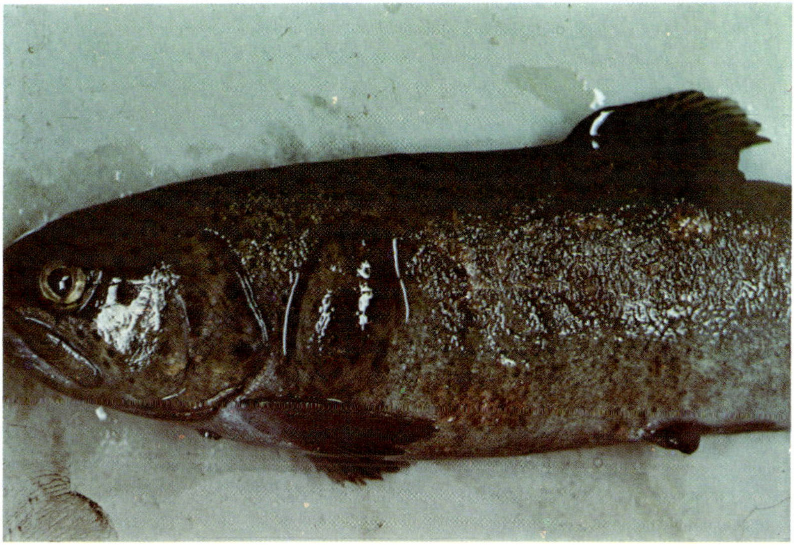

Figure 25. External symptoms of kidney disease in rainbow trout (*Salmo gairdneri*). Note the small ulcers.

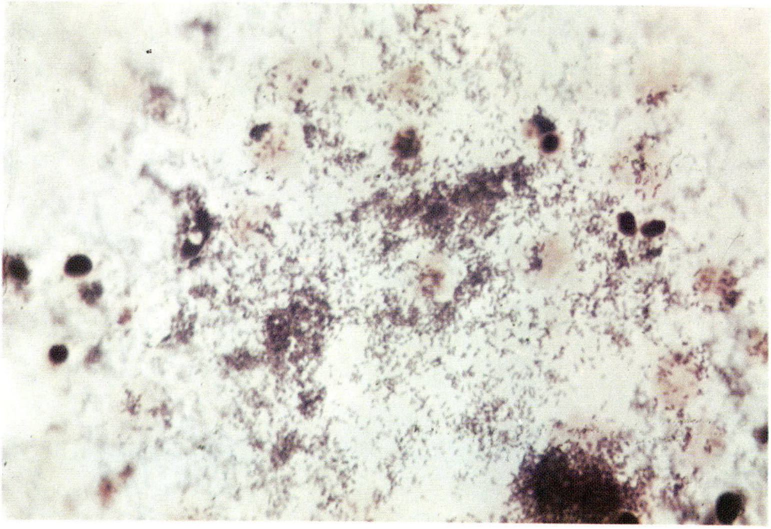

Figure 26. Photomicrograph of stained brook trout (*Salvelinus fontinalis*) kidney smear showing corynebacteria causing kidney disease (note intracellular forms. ×1000.

(See page 96)

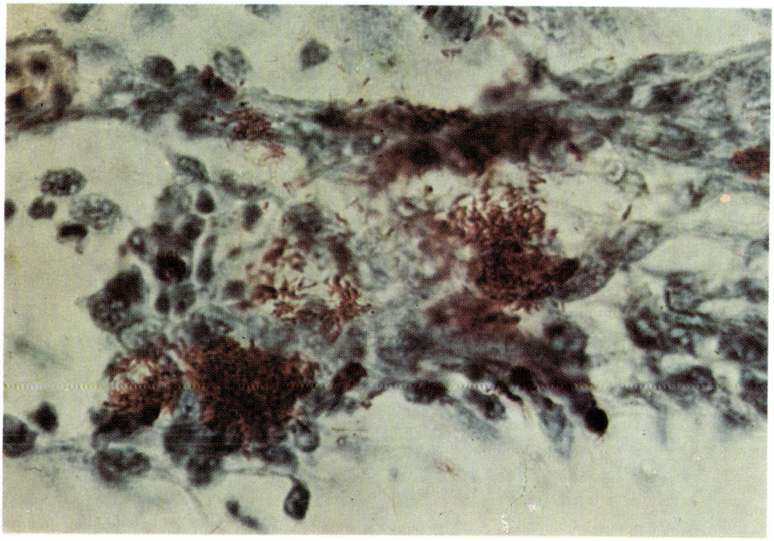

Figure 31. Acid fast stain of chinook salmon (*Oncorhynchus tshawytscha*) gill tissue showing mycobacteria.

(See page 107)

# The Identification of Fish Pathogenic Bacteria

by
Graham L. Bullock

Bureau of Sport Fisheries and Wildlife
Eastern Fish Disease Laboratory
Kearneysville, West Virginia 25430

## CONTENTS

## INTRODUCTION

Determining the identity of fish pathogenic bacteria is necessary for disease diagnosis, because some of the bacterial fish diseases, though caused by taxonomically different bacteria, have similar symptoms. Therefore correct diagnosis is not possible without identification of the etiologic agent and is also a necessary prerequisite to effective control because there are different control measures for different diseases.

The methods and procedures needed for identification of the bacteria causing common diseases of fishes are described in this chapter. If a particular disease is caused by an uncommon, or so far not recognized bacterium, special identification procedures described in textbooks of diagnostic or determinative bacteriology will have to be used.

Before bacteriological examination of fishes is started the diagnostician ought to have a clear understanding of the limitations of the methods and interpretation of the findings.

It is a well known fact that bacteria are present, often in large numbers, on the body surface and in the intestines of fish. It is also known that in fish which are considered healthy, saprophytic and pathogenic bacteria may be present in the bloodstream and internal organs but without causing disease (Bisset, 1948; Evelyn and McDermott, 1961; Bullock and Snieszko, 1969; Allan and Pelczar, 1967). Temperature and other environmental factors may increase considerably the incidence of systemic bacteria (Bisset, 1946) and the differences between infection without disease, and infection causing disease are rather tenuous. For this reason anyone performing bacteriological examination of fish in order to diagnose a disease ought to be thoroughly familiar with Koch's postulates and their interpretation.

In general, one seldom has a reason for bacteriological examination of fishes unless their behavior or appearance indicates that they are diseased. Since saprophytic bacteria which may be unrelated to the disease quickly penetrate bodies of dead fishes, diseased moribund specimens are most suitable for bacteriological examination. Healthy appearing fish in the same population should be examined simultaneously. If a certain type of bacterium is consistently present in external lesions or internal organs of diseased fishes and absent in healthy fishes one is justified in suspecting that this organism is the etiologic agent of the disease. If the bacterium isolated from the diseased fish is known to be a fish pathogen, and if some symptoms of the disease are typical, there is a well founded reason to accept the isolated bacterium as the true etiologic agent.

It is also possible that fish may be infected with two or more species of bacteria of which only one can be easily isolated and identified. In such case only a partially correct diagnosis is made. The diagnostician must also be aware of the probability that the primary cause of the disease may be a virus and the bacterium causes a superinfection. Therefore interpretation of bacteriological findings is not always a simple process and requires experience in fish pathology.

## METHODS OF EXAMINATION

The method used to identify a fish pathogen will vary with the particular disease. For example, gill disease or columnaris disease may be diagnosed by examination of a wet mount of affected material, while kidney disease is diagnosed on the basis of simple or gram stain. However, identification of furunculosis, hemorrhagic septicemia, and other diseases caused by closely related bacteria requires isolation and identification of the pathogen.

Examination of moribund fish may be accomplished by killing the specimen by exposure to strong anaesthetic, followed by disinfection, either by immersion or swabbing the body surface. If material from an open lesion is to be examined, immersion in a disinfectant should be avoided. After disinfection, the fish is placed in a freshly disinfected dissecting tray and covered with a paper towel moistened with disinfectant. The towel is removed, and, using sterilized or disinfected instruments, the fish is opened along the ventral surface and a part of the abdominal wall is removed to expost the internal organs with care taken not to damage them (Fig. 1). The

Figure 1. Rainbow trout opened ventrally to expose viscera and kidney for observation of pathology and/or bacteriological examination.

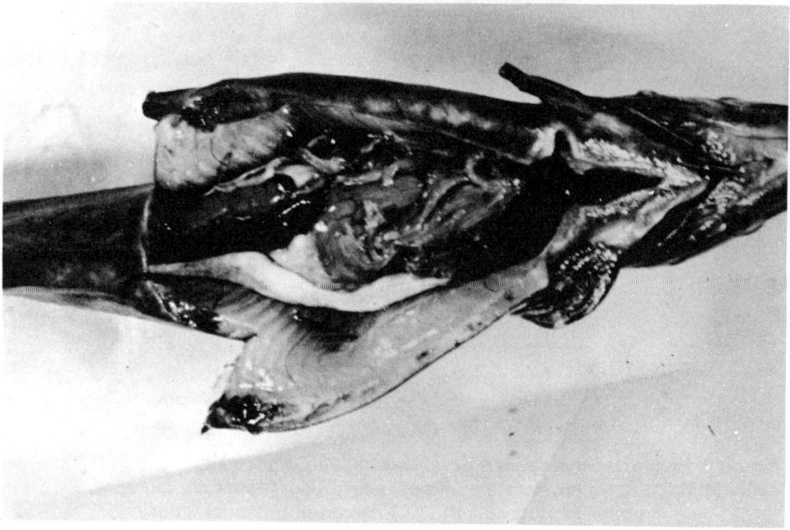

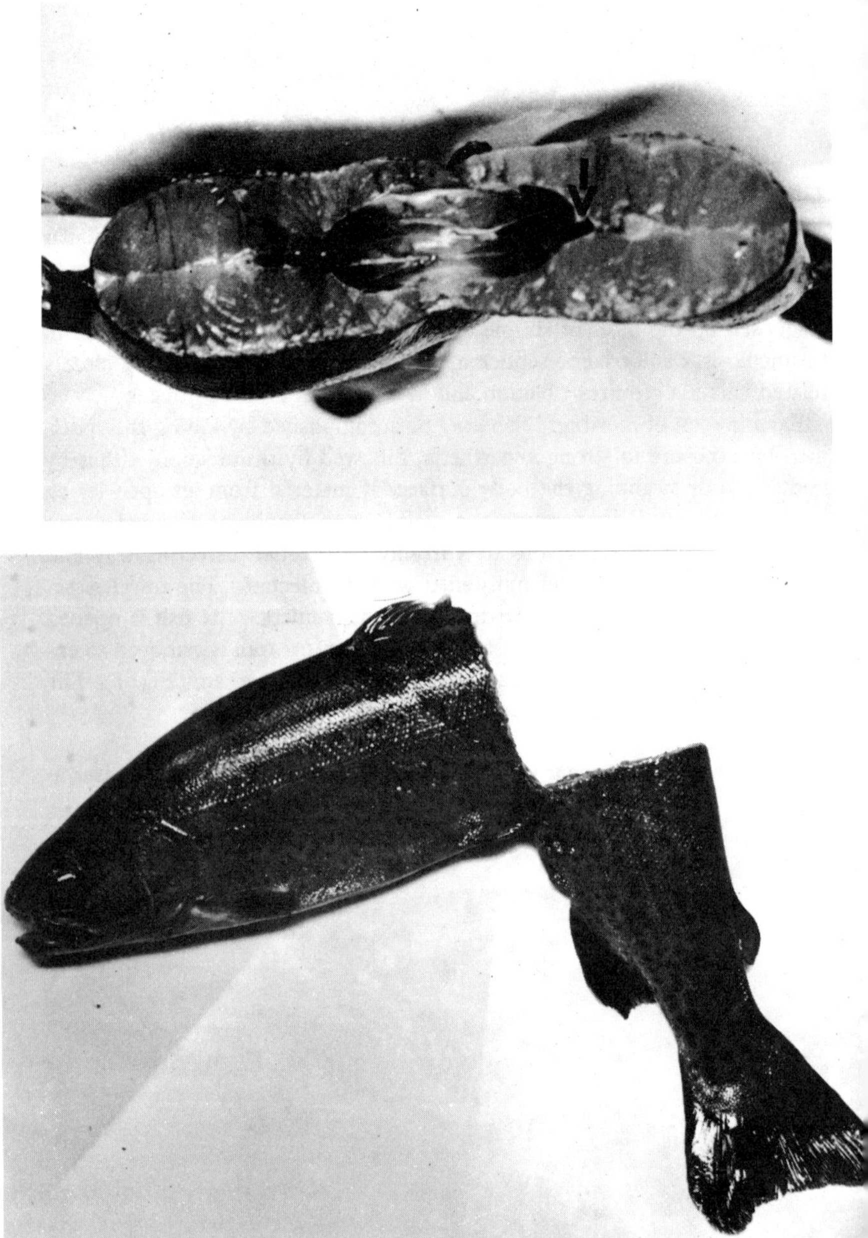

Figure 2. Rainbow trout opened dorso-ventrally to expose kidney for inoculation of bacteriological medium. Note that intestine is not cut (upper photograph). Arrow in upper photograph shows location of posterior kidney.

knowledge of the location of the internal organs in different species of fishes is necessary in order to make the incision in the right place. The internal pathology may be noted and material for staining and inoculation of media may be obtained from the organs. If the disease is septicemic, many of the internal organs are suitable for microscopic and bacteriological examination. As a general rule the kidney is usually used, but again this will vary with the fish under examination. Another way of obtaining material from the kidney in certain fishes, such as salmonids, is to make a cross cut behind the dorsal fin which extends through the muscle, kidney, backbone and into the peritoneal cavity, but not into the gut. The kidney is exposed and material may be obtained for examination by inserting an inoculating loop into the exposed portions of the kidney (Fig. 2). Material for cultures is usually streaked on media in petri plates which are then incubated at 20°–22°C (unless it is known other temperatures are more appropriate) until growth appears. If the growth consists of only one colony type, transfer is made from a well-separated colony to an agar slant or to any other selected media. If however more than one colony type is present each type would have to be restreaked for purity testing since only pure cultures are suitable for identification.

Among the procedures used in identifying the bacteria, the following are most important: determination of the cell morphology and staining characteristics; appearance of the colony; determination of physiological reactions; and serological typing. The appropriate method will be listed for each pathogen and will consist of key morphological and biochemical characteristics followed by serological procedures, if they have been developed for the particular pathogen. The serological procedures used so far consist of agglutination and precipitation tests. The use of direct or indirect fluorescent antibody technique has been used very little and then to demonstrate serotypes of *A. salmonicida* (Klontz and Anderson, 1968). Increased application of this technique will be helpful for diagnostic procedure.

Serotyping of each group of fish pathogenic bacteria is certainly possible and desirable by use of somatic, flagellar and capsular antigens. The serological procedures considered here will concern agglutination or agar gel precipitation tests by means of which species within a genus can be identified. Methods to be discussed are intended for identification of the most commonly encountered and typical fish pathogenic bacteria.

Formulations of stains, media, chemicals, and performance of diagnostic procedures are described in the appendix.

The flow charts (Figs. 3 and 4) give some of the differential characteristics used in identification of the important types of fish pathogenic bacteria. Explanations and procedures are given in the text.

## IDENTIFICATION OF GRAM-NEGATIVE BACTERIA

As it is evident from the flow charts (Figs. 3 and 4) the gram-negative bacteria cause a larger number of diseases than gram-positive bacteria and the former will be discussed first.

### Gram-negative non-motile rods

To this group belong *Aeromonas salmonicida* causing fish furunculosis, *Hemophilus piscium* causing ulcer disease, and *Flavobacterium* sp. causing poorly defined infections in freshwater and marine fishes.

1. *Aeromonas salmonicida* (furunculosis)
   a. Key morphological and biochemical characteristics.

      Gram-negative, non-motile rod 1.0 by 1.7–2.0 microns.

      Cytochrome oxidase positive.

      Produces brown water-soluble pigment in 48 hrs. or gives a positive paraphenylene diamine test after 24 hrs. incubation.

      Ferments o/f glucose with slight gas production.

      Typical brown pigment is produced best in cultures grown on trypticase soy agar (TSA) or furunculosis agar (FA).

   b. Serological diagnosis

      A slide agglutination test has been developed for rapid identification of *A. salmonicida* (Rabb, Cornick and McDermott, 1964).

2. *Hemophilus piscium* (ulcer disease)
   a. Key morphological and biochemical characteristics.

      Gram-negative, non-motile, rod .5–1.0 by 1.0–2.0 microns.

      Will not grow on TSA or FA but will grow on medium #8 plus fish peptone or on Mueller-Hinton medium (Difco) with cocarboxylase.

   b. Serological diagnosis

      Preliminary evidence indicates that a slide agglutination test is reliable and at present offers the most accurate method of identification (Bullock, unpublished data).

      The bacterium is found only in salmonids, particularly brook trout.

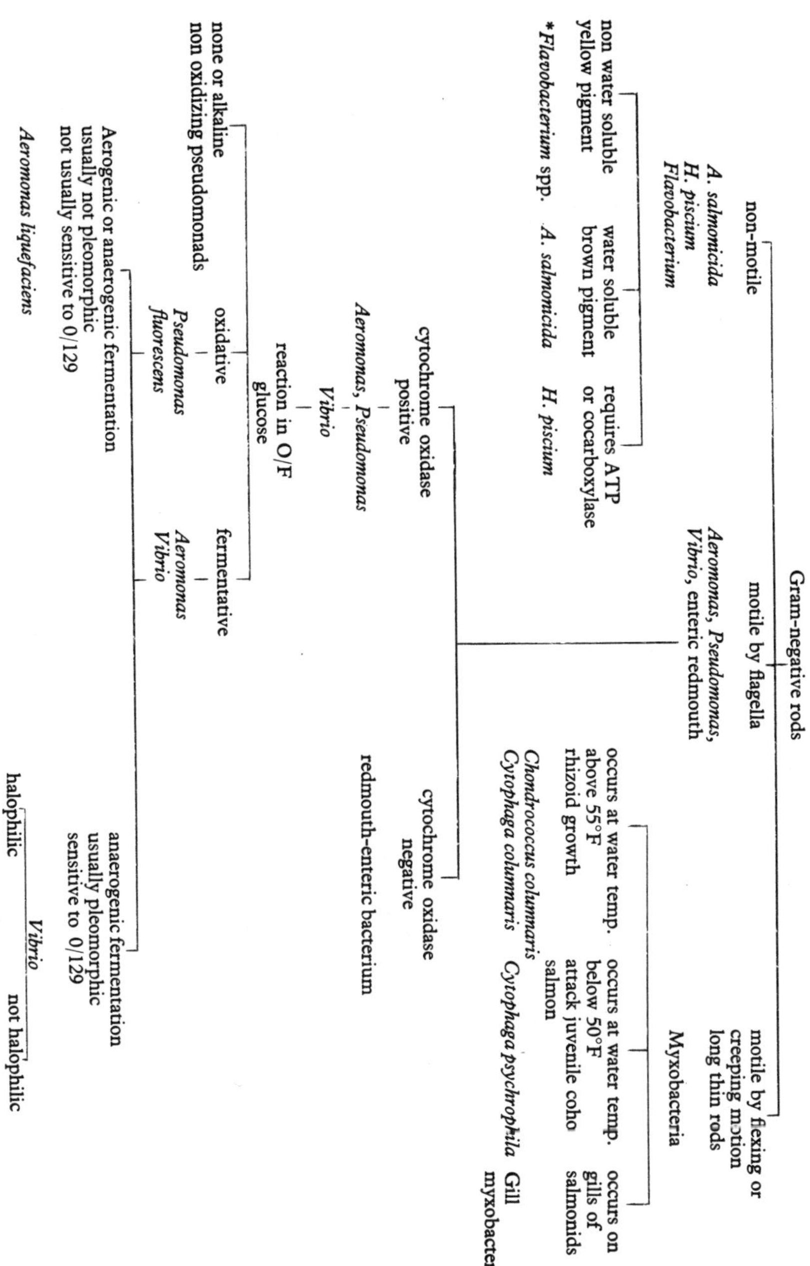


Figure 3. Differentiation of the most common gram-negative fish pathogenic bacteria.

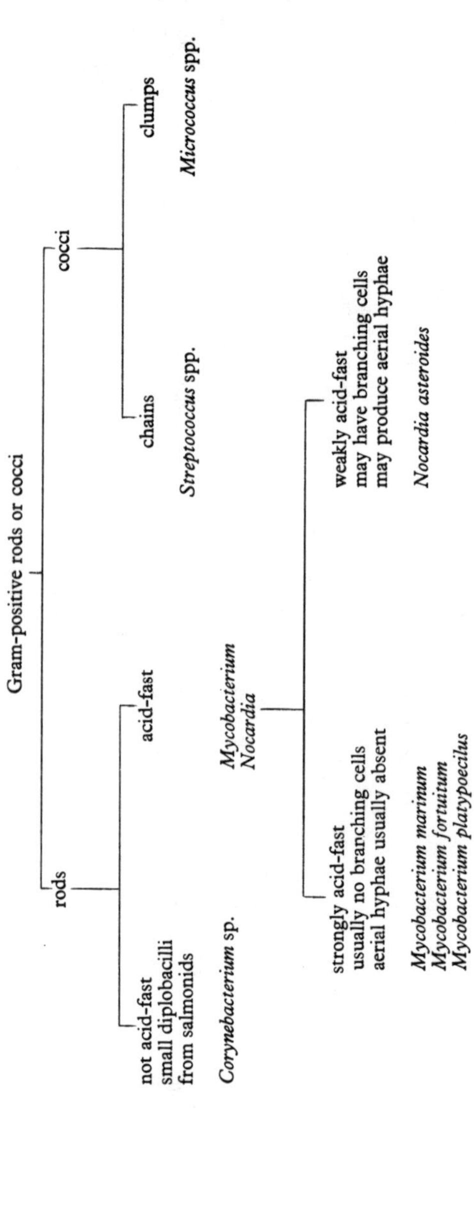


**Figure 4. Differentiation of most common gram-positive fish pathogenic bacteria.**

3. *Flavobacterium* sp.
   a. Key morphological and biochemical characteristics.
      Gram-negative, usually non-motile rod .5–1.0 by 1.0–3.0 microns.
      Some species may have peritrichous flagella.
      Produces yellow-orange water insoluble pigment.
      Grows on TSA or FA.
      Some are marine species requiring addition of NaCl (1.0–1.5 percent) to the medium.
      Flavobacteria may be differentiated from yellow pigmented myxobacteria by their inability to spread on media with reduced nutrient and agar.
      The above description is only a tentative identification to the genus. While *F. piscicida* is a recognized fish pathogen recent investigations indicate this bacterium belongs in the genus *Pseudomonas* (Buck, Meyers and Leifson, 1963).
   b. Serological diagnosis
      None at present.

**Gram-negative rods motile by polar flagella**

This group includes *Aeromonas liquefaciens* (synonyms: *A. punctata*, *A. hydrophila*) considered as the agent, or co-agent, of hemorrhagic septicemia (also infectious dropsy, or the German "Bauchwassersucht"); *Pseudomonas fluorescens* and other related pseudomonads such as *P. putida* and non-oxidizing pseudomonads all of which are involved in external or systemic fish infections; *Vibrio anguillarum* causing hemorrhagic septicemia in eels and other saltwater and brackish water fishes; *Vibrio parahaemolyticus*, a serious human pathogen in Japan and also occasionally a fish pathogen; and *Vibrio piscium* var. *japonicus* causing infections in freshwater fishes in Japan.

1. *A. liquefaciens* (hemorrhagic septicemia)
   a. Key morphological and biochemical characteristics.
      Gram-negative rod .75 by 1.0–1.5 microns.
      Motile by polar flagellum.
      Good growth on TSA, FA.
      Cytochrome oxidase positive.
      Aerogenic or anaerogenic fermentation of o/f glucose medium.
   b. Serological diagnosis
      Most of the strains so far tested formed precipitin bands with antisera prepared from *A. liquefaciens* cell extract material (Bullock, 1966).

2. *P. fluorescens* (hemorrhagic septicemia)
   a. Key morphological and biochemical characteristics.
      Gram-negative rod 0.5 by 1.0–2.0 microns.
      Motile by polar flagella (rarely non-motile, see Bullock, 1965).
      Good growth on TSA, FA
      Cytochrome oxidase positive.
      Oxidation of o/f glucose medium.
      Usually produces fluorescent pigment on *Pseudomonas F* agar slants.
   b. Serological diagnosis.
      None developed.
      At times organisms with characteristics similar to *P. fluorescens*, except that no reaction or an alkaline reaction occurs in o/f glucose medium, may be isolated from diseased fish. These bacteria have been called non-oxidizing pseudomonads. However further investigation may reveal they represent other genera and species.

3. *Vibrio anguillarum* (red pest of saltwater eels)
   a. Key morphological and biochemical characteristics.
      Gram-negative curved (not spiral) or straight rod 0.5 by 1.0–2.0 microns).
      Motile by polar flagella.
      Grow on FA, TSA with 1–1.5% sea salts or on the medium of Simidu and Hasu (1968a).
      Cytochrome oxidase positive.
      Anaerogenic fermentation of o/f or m-o-f glucose.
      Ferments celliobiose within 24 hrs. (Sakazaki, Iwanami and Fukumi, 1963).
      Sensitive to 0/129 vibriostatic agent.
   b. Serological diagnosis
      None at present.

4. *V. parahaemolyticus* (enteritis in human beings, septicemias in fishes)
   a. Key morphological and biochemical characteristics.
      Cell morphology similar to *V. anguillarum* and *A. liquefaciens*.
      Growth medium similar to *V. anguillarum*.
      Cytochrome oxidase positive.
      Anaerogenic fermentation of o/f glucose.
      Grows in broth medium with 7% NaCl (Sakazaki *et al.*, 1963).
      Will not ferment celliobiose in 24 hrs. (Sakazaki *et al.*, 1963).
      Sensitive to 0/129.
   b. Serological diagnosis
      Serotyping of strains.

5. *V. piscium* var. *japonicus* (Hoshina, 1957, furunculo-septicemia in Japanese rainbow trout; Saito, Otsuro, Furukawa, Kanda and Sato, 1964).
   a. Key morphological and biochemical characteristics.
      Because of cell curvature and other reactions, this bacterium is considered to belong to the *Vibrio* genus (Shewan, 1963). However it differs from the previous *Vibrio* by not requiring NaCl or sea water for growth, therefore it would be considered one of the freshwater vibrios.
   b. Serological diagnosis
      Twelve strains of *V. piscium* var. *japonicus* were found to be serologically identical but different from *V. comma* and other vibrios (Saito *et al.*, 1964). Presumably a slide agglutination test would be applicable.

**General comments on gram-negative polar flagellated rods**

Cell curvature in vibrios may vary to the extent that it is not of diagnostic value resulting in vibrio cultures being confused with anaerogenic aeromonads. This may be overcome by using either the vibriostatic agent 0/129 or testing the isolate for precipitin bands using *A. liquefaciens* antiserum. *A. liquefaciens* is not usually sensitive to 0/129 while the vibrios are; however, the 0/129 vibriostat is not available commercially. In tests using crude antigens, 60 out of 62 aerogenic and anaerogenic motile aeromonads formed precipitin bands with *A. liquefaciens* antiserum while the vibrio cultures isolated from fish did not (Bullock, 1966).

The following test may be of diagnostic value to differentiate further the anaerogenic aeromonads from vibrio species (Sakazaki *et al.*, 1963; Davis and Park, 1962).

| | Grow at pH 9-9.4 | Cells usually pleomorphic | Hydrolyze chitin | Growth on salmonella shigella agar |
|---|---|---|---|---|
| Anaerogenic aeromonads | − | − | − | + |
| Vibrio | + | + | + | − |

**Gram-negative rods motile by means of peritrichous flagella and cytochrome oxidase negative**

The only bacterium presently in this group is an unspeciated enteric bacterium causing redmouth in trout in the western United States. Ross, Rucker and Ewing (1966) suggested the temporary designation RM until the bacterium is named.

1. RM bacterium (redmouth)
   a. Key morphological and biochemical characteristics.
      The biochemical, morphological and some serological characteristics may be found in the study by Ross, Rucker and Ewing (1966).

The bacterium grows well on TSA and FA and may be separated from fermentative aeromonads and vibrios on the basis of both the cytochrome oxidase test and the peritrichous flagellation. The fact that the bacterium is found only in a few western states is also of diagnostic value.

b. Serological diagnosis

Identification of several strains of the organism has been accomplished with a rapid slide agglutination test using rabbit antiserum prepared from one strain (McDaniel, 1968, pers. comm.).

**Long, thin, gram-negative rods producing yellow pigmented colonies, motile by means of creeping or flexing motion**

Bacteria with these characteristics are classified as myxobacteria and the fish pathogenic forms are: *Chondrococcus columnaris* and *Cytophaga columnaris* causing columnaris disease; *Cytophaga psychrophila* causing coldwater (peduncle) disease; non-classified myxobacteria associated with gill diseases; and non-classified myxobacteria occurring in tail rot of salmonids.

1. *Chondrococcus columnaris* (columnaris disease)

a. Key morphological and biochemical characteristics.

Gram-negative aerobic rod .4–.8 micron wide by 2–12 microns long.

Motile by means of flexing or creeping.

Flat, spreading, irregular colonies on media with reduced agar content (1–1.1%).

Dry rhizoid growth which tends to adhere to solid media (Fig. 5).

Under specific conditions (Borg, 1948, 1960) *Chondrococcus columnaris* forms microcysts and fruiting bodies while *Cytophaga columnaris* does not and apparently this is the only major difference between these two myxobacteria.

Usually do not attack fish when water temperature is below 12°C.

b. Serological diagnosis

A slide agglutination test is applicable for identification of *Chondrococcus columnaris* because strains of *C. columnaris* possess a common antigen (Anacker and Ordal, 1955) and are also serologically distinct from other fish pathogenic myxobacteria (Bullock and McDaniel, unpublished).

Often many strains of *C. columnaris* when grown on either solid medium or in broth will produce rough cell suspensions which are unsuitable for agglutination tests. Smooth cell suspensions may be prepared by growing cultures in liquid Ordal's medium followed by centrifugation. The cells are then suspended in physiological saline and heated for 5 minutes at 50°C (Anacker and Ordal, 1955).

2. *Cytophaga psychrophila* (coldwater or peduncle disease)
   a. Key morphological and biochemical characteristics.
   Gram-negative aerobic rod .75 micron wide by 3.5–7.5 microns long. Produce moist, yellow pigmented colonies on Ordal's agar (Fig. 5) which spread slowly. They produce neither fruiting bodies nor microcysts and usually cause disease in fish at water temperature below 10°C, ideally at 5°–7°C.
   b. Serological diagnosis
   Preliminary evidence indicates that a rapid slide agglutination test is specific for *C. psychrophila* (Pacha, 1968; Bullock and McDaniel, unpublished).
3. Gill disease myxobacteria (bacterial gill disease)
   a. Key morphological and biochemical characteristics.
   Although there are serological similarities among myxobacterial strains isolated from outbreaks of gill disease, no one has shown that either one or several species are involved in gill disease of cultured salmonids. The characteristics of pure cultures of myxobacteria so far isolated from the gills of trout with gill disease are as follows:
   Gram-negative, aerobic rods 0.5 wide by 4.5–5.0 microns, which produce light yellow moist spreading colonies on Ordal's agar (Fig. 5).

Figure 5. Colonial morphology of three fish pathogenic myxobacteria, grown 72 hours on cytophage agar:
A. *Chondrococcus columnaris*, colony diameter 12mm.
B. *Cytophaga psychrophila*, colony diameter 5 mm.
C. Gill disease myxobacterium, colony diameter 25mm.

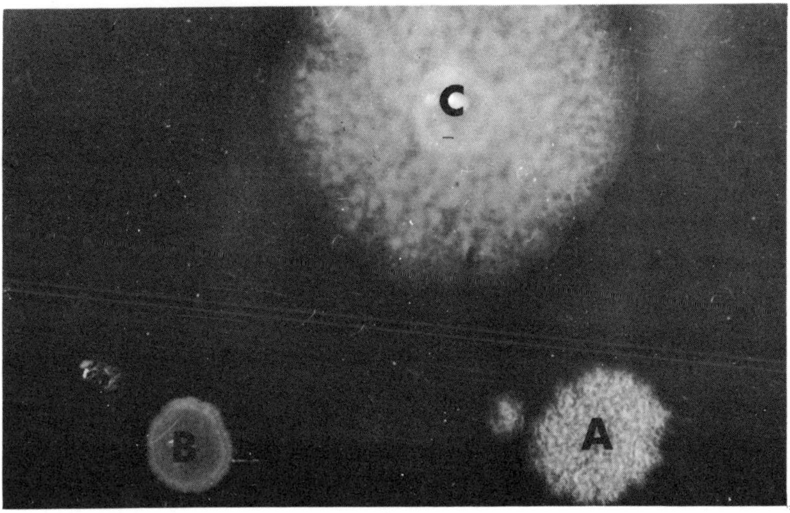

They have not been observed to form microcysts or fruiting bodies therefore they should be classified as *Cytophaga*.
There is no evidence that gill disease myxobacteria cause systemic infections.

b. Serological diagnosis
   None at present.

4. Tail and fin rot myxobacteria
   a. Key morphological and biochemical characteristics
      Myxobacteria isolated from fin and tail rot lesions, especially in cultured salmonids, constitute a diversified unclassified *Cytophaga*-like species. Their role in tail and fin rot is not established but they produce severe lesions once they infect the tissue.
   b. Serological diagnosis
      None at present.

## IDENTIFICATION OF GRAM-POSITIVE BACTERIA

As previously discussed, there are fewer gram-positive than gram-negative fish pathogenic bacteria. Among them are the kidney disease corynebacterium, mycobacteria, and occasionally isolated streptococci and microcci.

### Gram-positive, non-motile, non-acid-fast rods

1. *Corynebacterium* sp. (kidney disease)
   a. Key morphological characteristics
      Gram-positive rod 0.3–0.5 micron wide by 0.5–1.0 micron long.
      Non-motile.
      Because this bacterium is difficult to grow, diagnosis is based on microscopic examination of material from lesions. While the presence of the typical kidney disease corynebacterium indicates infection, the severity of this disease depends on the size and numbers of lesions. Light infections do not cause visible disease symptoms or mortalities (Fig. 6). If isolation of the kidney disease bacterium is undertaken, the

Figure 6. Kidney smear of trout that died from kidney disease. Note the massive numbers of Corynebacteria.

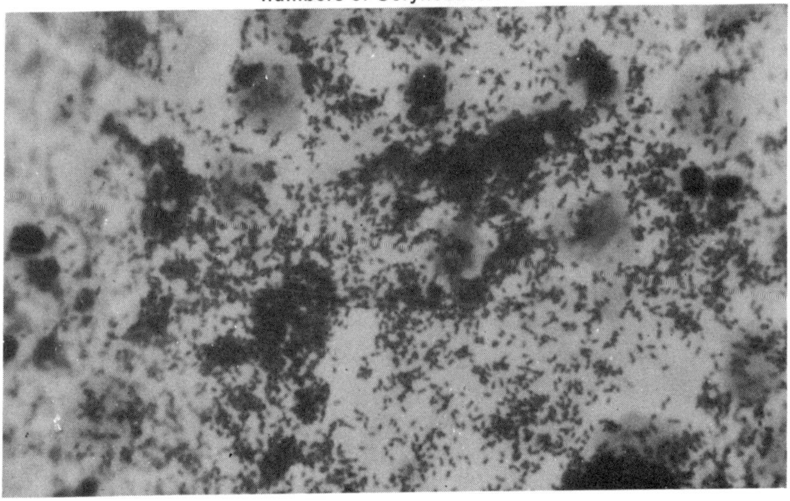

media of Ordal and Earp (1956) or Smith's (1964) modification of the same medium, is recommended.

b. Serological diagnosis

None at present.

**Gram-positive, non-motile, non-acid-fast Cocci**

1. Cells occur in chains.

   *Streptococcus* sp.

2. Cells occur in irregular clumps.

   *Micrococcus* sp.

Since gram-positive cocci rarely cause disease in fishes, little information exists as to diagnostic methods of identification. However a recent epizootic among catfish was caused by a *Streptococcus* sp. (Robinson and Meyer, 1966). If cocci are encountered as disease agents of fishes, the reader is referred to *Manual for the Identification of Medical Bacteria* by Cowan and Steele (1965) as an aid in identification.

**Gram-positive, non-motile, acid-fast rods**

1. Mycobacterium

   *M. marinum*, *M. fortuitum*, *M. platypoecilis* } fish mycobacteriosis

   a. Key morphological and biochemical characteristics

      Gram-positive generally non-branching rods, usually 1.0–3.0 microns long but may appear as long thin beaded or barred rods.

      Aerial hyphae usually not produced.

      Non-motile.

      Acid-fast.

      Aerobic.

      Sugars are attacked by oxidation.

      The listed species are the only fish pathogens recognized in the 7th Edition of *Bergey's Manual* (Breed, Murray and Smith, 1957). Differentiation of species may be difficult. Information listed in Table 1 may be helpful, but positive identification at the species level should be made by someone familiar with mycobacteria from cold-blooded vertebrates.

   b. Serological diagnosis

      None at present.

2. *Nocardia asteroides*—at present this species is the only one reported to be pathogenic for fishes.

   a. Key morphological characteristics

      Gram-positive, branching rods.

      Non-motile.

Aerobic.

Weakly acid-fast when stained in tissues, but cultures may not be acid-fast.

Aerial hyphae may be produced.

Vegetative mycelium fragments into branched or unbranched rods which are generally longer than mycobacterial cells, but this cannot always be relied upon to differentiate the two genera.

*Nocardia* species usually grow within 2–3 days and therefore may be confused with *M. fortuitum*, but usually not the slower growing fish pathogenic mycobacteria. *Nocardia* sp. may also be confused with species in the genus *Streptomyces*. Since *Nocardia* species have properties similar to both *Mycobacterium* and *Streptomyces*, it is possible the *Nocardia* represent a transition between *Mycobacterium* and *Streptomyces* which would in part explain the difficulty in identification of *Nocardia*.

For more information on the systematics of mycobacteria the papers by Bojalil and Cerbon (1961); Gordon (1966); Jones and Jenkins (1965); Manion, Bradley, Zinneman and Hall (1964); Sherris (1963) may be helpful. Also the papers by Gordon and Mihm (1957, 1962); Adams and McClung (1960, 1962) and Zamora, Bojalil and Bastarrachea (1963) give some current views on taxonomy of *Nocardia*.

TABLE 1. Characteristics of acid-fast bacilli isolated from fish and recognized by *Bergey's Manual* (7th Edition, Breed *et al.*, 1957) (Parisot, 1958, Modified).

| | *Mycobacterium fortuitum* | *Mycobacterium marinum* | *Mycobacterium platypoecilis* |
|---|---|---|---|
| Morphology | Acid-fast, gram-positive, non-motile, slender rods occasionally beaded | Acid-fast, gram-positive, non-motile, pleomorphic, banded or beaded rods | Acid-fast, gram positive, straight rods; not as pleomorphic as the human bacillus |
| Cultural characteristics: | | | |
| (a) Media | Glycerol agar, Dorset's medium, Heart Infusion Broth | Glycerol agar, Heart Infusion Broth, Petroff's medium | Glycerolated egg, glycerine phosphate, Sohngen's medium |
| (b) temperature | 28-35°C. Grow at 40°C. Not survive 65°C for 4 hrs. | 18-20°C. No growth at 47°C. Killed at 60°C for 1 hr. | 25°C. No growth at 37°C. Temperature range not investigated thoroughly. |
| (c) Growth time | 3-4 days on agar | 14-18 days on agar; grew more rapidly when sub-cultured | 3 weeks on glycerolated agar. |

| | | | |
|---|---|---|---|
| (d) Colony characteristics | 14 days glycerol agar; off-white to beige color. Growth abundant, spreading, glistening or dull, rough and waxy | Smooth, moist, elevated, lemon-yellow to deep orange in old cultures | Smooth and moist when young. Rough and dried when old. Deep orange color when cultured in light |
| Pathogenicity | Neon tetra. Not pathogenic for rabbits, mice or guinea pigs | Frogs, mice, pigeons, salt-water fish. Not for rabbits or guinea pigs | Mexican platyfish. Not for goldfish. No other animals tested |
| Source | Soil, infections in humans and coldblooded animals | Sea bass, croaker, Sergeant major, saltwater fish | Mexican platyfish, warmwater fish |

## BACTERIA RARELY ENCOUNTERED AS FISH PATHOGENS

The foregoing discussion of gram-positive and gram-negative bacteria which are pathogenic to fishes, represents the types usually encountered. Significant outbreaks of fish diseases caused by bacteria not covered in the discussion have occurred, as for example, the white perch epizootic caused by *Pasteurella piscicida* (Snieszko, Bullock, Hollis and Boone, 1964; Janssen and Surgalla, 1968) and may be expected to occur. This emphasizes the fact that any diagnostic key is incomplete and serves as an aid in identification of only the most common pathogens. When fish pathogenic bacteria are isolated which do not fit in the scheme, additional characteristics of the isolate will have to be determined in order to identify the bacterium, using *Bergey's Manual of Determinative Bacteriology* (Breed *et al.*, 1957) or *Guide to the Identification of the Genera of Bacteria* (Skerman, 1967). If the taxonomic position is still not clear then it is possible the isolate represents an undescribed genus and species as in the case of the enteric bacterium causing redmouth in rainbow trout in the western United States (Ross *et al.*, 1966).

## STAINS, MEDIA AND METHODS USED IN IDENTIFICATION OF FISH PATHOGENIC BACTERIA

The material presented below is intended as an aid to identification procedures. Since the methods, media and stains given are limited to those used most frequently, additional procedures may be found in the *Manual of Microbiological Methods* (Society of American Bacteriologists, 1957); *A Guide to the Identification of the Genera of Bacteria* (Skerman, 1967); *Identification of Medical Bacteria* (Cowan and Steel, 1965), as well as the methods listed in the manuals of manufacturers of bacteriological media.

Most of the materials listed below are available from scientific supply houses. In case of rarely used materials, sources are given.

### Stains

*Staining of bacteria in fixed smears*

1. Clean slide with non-scratching cleaning powder.
2. When dry, wipe off the cleaning material.
3. Spread the material on the slide.
   a. Take a small particle of tissue, blood, or secretion and spread it evenly on a slide by means of a scalpel or clean inoculating loop.
   b. If material is too dry, add a drop of clean water.
   c. Another way is to put material on one slide and mash with another, slide slides apart and stain one or both.
4. When air-dry fix by pouring methyl alcohol over slide, leave for one minute and let evaporate or burn off. Another common way of fixing is by passing a slide over a flame but this is not considered an equally good method.
5. Use desired staining procedure (simple,gram, etc.).
6. Wash with clean tap (or distilled) water.
7. Let dry completely (one can use a blotter).
8. Examine under the microscope using oil immersion lens.

*Simple stain procedures*

1. Prepare smear on a slide as thin as practicable and air-dry.
2. Fix with methyl alcohol or in flame.
3. Stain for 5–30 seconds.
4. Wash in water 5–10 seconds.
5. Blot off excess water and air-dry.

*Simple stain solutions*

1. Pinacyanolchloride

| | | |
|---|---|---|
| Pinacyanolchloride (Eastman Kodak) | 0.25 | g |
| 70% methyl or ethyl alcohol | 100 | ml |

(Prior fixing is not required with this stain).

2. Methylene blue (Loeffler)

Solution A

| | | |
|---|---|---|
| Methylene blue (90% dye content) | 0.3 | g |
| Ethyl alcohol (95%) | 30 | ml |

Solution B

| | | |
|---|---|---|
| Diluted KOH (0.01% by weight) | 100 | ml |

Mix solutions A and B.

*Gram's method of staining* (Hucker's modification)

1. Prepare slide in the usual manner.
2. Fix with methyl alcohol or in flame.
3. Flood with crystal violet for one minute.
4. Rinse in tap water, do not extend for more than 5 seconds.
5. Cover with iodine solution for 20–30 seconds.
6. Rinse well with tap water (5–10 seconds).
7. Decolorize for about 30 seconds with 95% ethyl alcohol plus 5% acetone (this step requires skill and experience).
8. Wash immediately with tap water and pour it off.
9. Counterstain for 10 seconds with safranin or for 20–30 seconds with carbol fuchsin diluted with distilled water 1:10.
10. Rinse in tap (or distilled) water.
11. Dry and examine.
    Gram-positive bacteria are dark-purple; the gram-negative are stained faintly pink or red.

*Solutions for gram stain*

1. Crystal violet

Solution A

| | | |
|---|---|---|
| Crystal violet | 2 | g |
| Ethyl alcohol | 20 | ml |

Solution B

| | | |
|---|---|---|
| Ammonium oxalate | 0.8 | g |
| Distilled water | 80 | ml |

Mix solution A and B.

2. Iodine solution

| | | |
|---|---|---|
| Iodine | 1 | g |
| Potassium iodide (KI) | 2 | g |
| Distilled water | 5 | ml |

When iodine is completely dissolved add 295 ml distilled water.

3. Safranin

| | | |
|---|---|---|
| Safranin 0 (2.5% in 95% ethyl alcohol) | 10 | ml |
| Distilled water | 100 | ml |

*Acid-fast staining*

1. Stain dried and fixed smears 3–5 minutes with Ziehl's carbol fuchsin applying enough heat for gentle steaming or bring to boiling.
2. Rinse in tap water.
3. Decolorize in 95% alcohol, containing 3% by volume of concentrated HCl, until only a suggestion of pink remains.
4. Wash in tap water.
5. Counterstain with methylene blue.
6. Wash in tap water.
7. Dry and examine.

   Acid-fast organisms are red; other bacteria and tissue material are blue.

*Solutions for acid-fast staining*

1. Carbol fuchsin (Ziehl's) for acid-fast

Solution A

| | | |
|---|---|---|
| Basic fuchsin | 0.3 | g |
| Ethyl alcohol (95%) | 10.0 | ml |

Solution B

| | | |
|---|---|---|
| Phenol | 5.0 | g |
| Distilled water | 95 | ml |

Mix solution A and B: for the staining of acid-fast bacteria use undiluted. For ordinary staining or for counterstaining in the Gram's method, dilute 1:10 with distilled water.

*Flagella staining* (Novel's method)

There are many methods of staining flagella and it is usually necessary for an individual to try several methods before finding one which consistently works. The procedure below has been used successfully for many years at the Eastern Fish Disease Laboratory.

Preparation of slides

1. Use new slides.
2. Clean with Bon Ami.
3. Flame side of slide to be used until flame around edges of slide shows traces of yellow.
4. Allow to cool thoroughly and then place slide in slanting position, with the flamed side face up.

Preparation of cell suspension

1. Use a 24 hr. culture and always check for motility, by hanging drop method before preparing suspension.
2. Use one of the following methods for preparation of cell suspension:

a. Formaldehyde method (Leifson, 1961).

Use a 24 hr. broth culture of organism to be stained. Add formalin (about 40% solution of formaldehydè) until the final concentration of formalin in the broth culture is 5–10%. Centrifuge formalized cells, pour off supernatant fluid, and resuspend packed cell pellet in distilled water. Centrifuge a second time and resuspend cells in 2–3 ml of distilled water.

b. Live cell suspension

By means of a platinum loop, gently suspend cells from a 24 hr. slant culture into 2–3 ml of distilled water. Allow the suspension to stand undisturbed for about 5–10 minutes.

Remarks: The use of formalin treated cell suspensions results in nice preparations, but sometimes the morphology of the flagella is changed by the addition of formalin. If critical morphological work is planned, then stains with live cell suspensions should be used first to check morphology of flagella. Also when using live cell suspensions, material should be drawn from the very top of the suspension to obtain free moving well dispersed cells.

Preparation of cells on slide

1. Allow 1–2 drops of cell suspension (from either a or b methods) to run down the middle of the previously flamed slanted slide. Allow material to air-dry, but *do not fix*.

*Staining* (Novel, 1939)

1. Mordant

Mix together: 50 ml of 20% tannic acid, 40 ml of cold saturated $FeSO_4 \cdot 7H_2O$, and 7 ml of saturated alcoholic solution of basic fuchsin or gentian violet. Allow mixture to stand for about 5 minutes and then filter onto slide. Stain for 1–1½ minutes and then rise well with distilled water.

2. Background

Add 10% ammonium hydroxide to about 20 ml of 5% silver nitrate until the brown precipitate disappears. Then add silver nitrate dropwise, until the solution is opalescent, but no precipitate is present. Pour onto slide and stain for 50–70 seconds, or until brown. Rinse well with distilled water, blot dry and examine.

## Media

For information on the general procedures of media preparation, the reader is referred to the *Manual of Microbiological Methods* (Society of American Bacteriologists, 1957).

## General laboratory media

Any medium which will support the growth of the non-fastidious pathogens such as *A. salmonicida*, *A. liquefaciens* or *P. fluorescens* may be used. The following are used routinely:

| | |
|---|---|
| Trypticase Soy Agar (BBL[1])<br>Furunculosis Agar (Difco[2]) | Prepare as directed on label. |

*Media for growing H. piscium*

Leetown Medium #8 plus fish peptone

| | | |
|---|---|---|
| Casitone or other tryptic digest of casein | 5 | g |
| Yeast extract | 5 | g |
| Sodium chloride | 5 | g |
| Maltose (technical) | 5 | g |
| Agar | 15 | g |
| Distilled water | 1000 | ml |

Combine ingredients in water, heat to boiling to dissolve agar, dispense in tubes or bottles and autoclave 15 minutes at 15 lbs. steam pressure. After sterilization, cool medium to 50°C and aseptically add 5% fish peptone. After addition of fish peptone, pour plates or prepare slants. *DO NOT* reheat medium once fish peptone has been added.

**Preparation of fish peptone**

1. Use one part brook trout tissue (whole fish but without stomach and gut) and two parts tap or distilled water.
2. Blend in a Waring blender for 1–2 minutes.
3. Add 1.5–2.0% (by volume) of concentrated hydrochloric acid and 1 gram per liter of powdered pepsin. Digest at 37–42°C for 12 hours stirring occasionally.
4. Adjust to pH 6.5 with 10–20% sodium hydroxide.
5. Transfer to a liter graduate cyclinder for settling. Add 1–2% (by volume) of chloroform and place in a refrigerator overnight or until particulate matter settles.
6. Siphon off supernatant fluid and filter sterilize.
7. Transfer aseptically to sterile tubes and add 1–2 milliliters of chloroform as preservative to each 20 milliliters of sterile fish peptone.

Simplified medium for *H. piscium*

Prepare Mueller-Hinton medium (Difco) as directed, autoclave and cool to 50°C. Aseptically add a solution of cocarboxylase as described below (thiamine pyrophosphate and diphosphothiamine are synonyms) at the rate of 5% to obtain the final concentration of 2 micrograms per milliliter of medium.

**Preparation of cocarboxylase**

Stock solution contains 0.1% cocarboxylase in distilled water and is sterilized by filtration. The stock solution may be stored several months in the refrigerator and is diluted 1:25 in sterile distilled water before use.

[1]Baltimore Biological Laboratories, Baltimore, Md.
[2]Difco Laboratories, Detroit, Michigan.

*Media for growing fish myxobacteria*

As a rule, media for myxobacteria contain reduced amounts of both nutrients and agar and most any medium which has been diluted to contain one-fifth to one-tenth the usual percentage of nutrients and one percent agar for solid media is suitable for use. The following media of Anacker and Ordal (1955) are most commonly used.

Solid:

| | |
|---|---|
| Tryptone | 0.5 g |
| Yeast extract | 0.5 g |
| Sodium acetate | 0.2 g |
| Beef extract | 0.2 g |
| Agar | 9.0 g (This has recently been increased to 11.0 g to facilitate streaking). |
| Distilled water | 1000 ml |
| pH 7.2 | |

Liquid:

| | |
|---|---|
| Tryptone | 4.0 g |
| Yeast infusion* | 30.0 ml |
| Tween 80 | 1.0 g |
| Water | 1000 ml |
| pH 7.2 | |

*Yeast infusion may be prepared by:

1. Suspend 10% by weight fresh baking yeast in tap water, autoclave 3 hrs. and let stand for several days.
2. Siphon off the supernatant, sterilize in screw cap tubes and store indefinitely (*Manual of Microbiological Methods*, 1957, p. 44).

Most fish myxobacteria will also grow on a simple medium containing 0.25% tryptone and 1.0% agar in tap or distilled water.

*Selective medium for myxobacteria*

The following medium described by Carlson and Pacha (1968) was effective in reducing growth of eubacteria and molds but not myxobacteria. Although the medium was designed to isolate myxobacteria from aquatic environments, it may be useful in isolating myxobacteria from diseased fish.

| | |
|---|---|
| Tryptone | 0.005% |
| Yeast extract | 0.005% |
| Sodium acetate | 0.002% |
| Beef extract | 0.002% |
| Peptonized milk | 0.05 % |
| Agar | 1.5 % |
| pH 6.8 | |

After autoclaving 20 minutes at 15 psi, 5 micrograms per milliliter of Neomycin and 10 micrograms per milliliter of cyclohexamide are added to the medium.

Before inoculation, plates are dried at 37°C for 48–72 hrs.

*Media for growing mycobacteria and nocardia*

Although many mycobacteria and nocardia species from fish will grow on TSA or FA, it is desirable to grow them, at least initially, on media specifically designed for them. One medium designed for isolation and maintenance of mycobacteria is Lowenstein-Jensen medium. This may be obtained commercially prepared, tubed and ready for use. Several other prepared media are also available from commercial supply houses.

*Medium for growth of the kidney disease bacterium*

The medium of Ordal and Earp (1956) has been and is now used to cultivate the kidney disease bacterium.

| | |
|---|---|
| Tryptose | 10.0 g |
| Beef extract | 3.0 g |
| NaCl | 5.0 g |
| Yeast extract | 0.5 g |
| Cysteine HCl | 1.0 g |
| Human blood | 200.0 ml |
| Agar | 15.0 g |
| Distilled water to make | 1000 ml |

Smith (1964) found that the substitution of horse blood for human blood also supported the growth of the kidney disease bacterium. Probably sterile blood of other animals would be equally satisfactory.

*Media for growing marine or estuarine fish pathogens*

Marine agar (Difco) prepared as directed is suitable for growing marine organisms, but bacteria from estuarine sources should have a reduced amount of salts (1.0–1.5%). This may be accomplished by making half strength marine agar and adding back nutrients and agar or by adding 1.2–1.5% of synthetic seawater salts (commercially available) to most any medium suitable for growth of freshwater forms.

Recent studies have indicated that bacteria from marine fish had different salt requirements than those from seawater (Simidu and Hasuo, 1968a) and an improved medium was given for isolation of bacteria from marine fish (Simidu and Hasuo, 1968b). The inorganic ions totaled about half that of seawater and the ionic ratio of sodium and potassium is nearly 1:1.

The composition of the medium is given below:

| | |
|---|---|
| Polypeptone (Daigo)[3] | 10.0 g |
| Lab Lemco (Oxoid)[4] | 3.0 g |
| Yeast extract (Difco) | 3.0 g |
| NaCl | 8.0 g |
| KCl | 10.0 g |

[3]Daigo Eiyo Kagaku Co., Osaka, Japan.

[4]Consolidated Laboratories Inc., Chicago Heights, Illinois, U.S.A.

| | |
|---|---|
| $MgSO4.7\ H_2O$ . . . . . . . . . . . . . | 3.0 g |
| $CaCl_2.\ 2\ H_2O$ . . . . . . . . . . . . . . | 1.5 g |
| Agar . . . . . . . . . . . . . . . . . . . . . | 12.0 g |
| Tap water . . . . . . . . . . . . . . . . . | 1000 ml |
| pH 7.5 | |

It is possible other high quality peptone may be substituted for polypeptone (Daigo) and beef extract used in place of Lab Lemco.

*Medium for chitin hydrolysis*

Trypticase Soy Agar plus 1.0% NaCl plus 10% chitin.

Examine daily for clear zones indicating breakdown of chitin.

*Media for Demonstration of Carbohydrate Utilization*

There are several types of basal media to which carbohydrates may be added. However in the diagnostic procedures as described, there is more need for the method showing how sugars are utilized, namely by oxidation or fermentation. For this purpose the Oxidation-Fermentation Basal Medium (o/f basal medium, Difco) or the Marine Oxidation Fermentation Basal Medium (m-o-f basal medium, Difco) are well suited. The media are prepared according to directions and the carbohydrate (usually glucose) is aseptically added to a final concentration of one percent.

*Method*

For each culture to be tested, two tubes of o/f glucose (or m-o-f glucose) are inoculated. After inoculation one of the two tubes is overlaid with sterile vaseline. Cultures are incubated and reactions recorded (or observed).

Figure 7. Oxidation and fermentation reactions in o/f glucose. The two tubes on the right show oxidation; the two tubes on the left show aerogenic fermentation. (This figure, reproduced in color, appears after Index.)

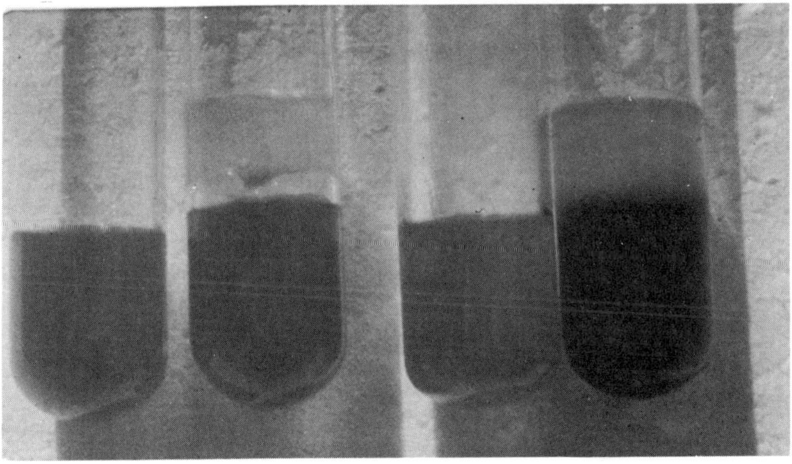

*Oxidation* (Fig. 7)

Before inoculation, medium was blue. After inoculation and incubation, color of tube without vaseline seal has turned to yellow indicating acid production and thus, glucose has been metabolized. Color of medium in sealed tube is still blue indicating glucose has not been attacked. This reaction is termed oxidation because the glucose was attacked only in the presence of air.

*Fermentation* (Fig. 7)

After incubation, color of medium in *both* tubes has turned to yellow showing that the glucose has attacked in the presence (open tube) or absence (closed tube) of air. Also the vaseline seal has been lifted indicating that acid and gas were produced from the glucose. Some fermentative organisms, however, do not form gas and the vaseline seal would remain in contact with the medium.

*No reaction or alkaline reaction*

Color of medium in both sealed and open tubes remain blue or color of medium in open tube becomes darker blue to purple due to release of ammonia from degradation of protein source in medium.

The reactions in m-o-f medium with glucose are interpreted in the same manner except that the color of uninoculated medium is pink.

*Detection of Fluorescent Pigment*

Many strains of *P. fluorescens* produce a fluorescent pigment and this is of diagnostic value. Prepare slants of Pseudomonas F Agar (Difco) and inoculate organism to be tested. Incubate at 20°–22°C for 24–48 hours and expose culture tube to ultraviolet light in a darkened room. If fluorescent pigment is present, the whole slant will "glow" or fluoresce under ultraviolet light, while an uninoculated slant will not.

## Other Diagnostic tests

1. Cytochrome oxidase test

This test is greatly simplified by the use of commercially available paper strips impregnated with the proper chemicals.[5]

Remove some growth with a platinum inoculating loop from a 24–48 hr. slant culture and spread thoroughly over one of the two reagent zones on the paper. If the test is positive a bright blue color develops within 1 minute (Fig. 8).

2. 0/129 Vibriostat[6] (2:4 diamino 6:7 DI isopropyl pteridine
2:4 diamino 6:7 DI isopropyl pteridine phosphate).

[5]PathoTec Co., General Diagnostics Division of Warner Chilcott, Morris Plains, N.J., U.S.A.

[6]This chemical is not commercially available but we have obtained 1 gram samples from the company: Allen and Hanburys, Ltd., Ware, Hertfordshire, England.

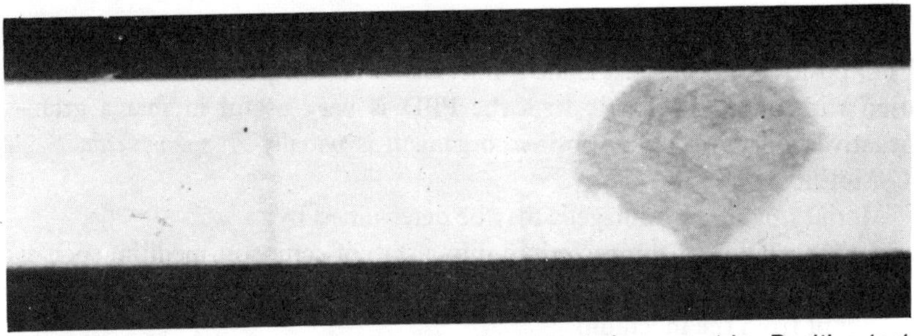

Figure 8. Cytochrome oxidase test using impregnated paper strip. Positive test indicated by blue color.
(This figure, reproduced in color, appears after Index.)

Only the phosphate derivative is water soluble, so Schubert (1962) developed the following procedure for using either form. His experiments had shown that 10 micrograms of 0/129 per disc were sufficient to show the desired results.

a. Prepare a 0.1 percent solution of the 0/129 phosphate form in water, or the 0/129 in Dioxan.[7]
b. Filter sterilize.
c. Add either solution to paper discs (7.0 millimeter) by pipetting .01 milliliter of solution per disc.
d. Dry discs.
e. Inoculate an agar slant by making a single streak from bottom to top of slant. Any medium which will support the growth of the organism is adequate for the 0/129 test.
f. Aseptically place a disc in the middle of streak and incubate culture at 20°–30°C for 24–48 hours.
g. Sensitive cultures (vibrios) will show a clear area on either side of the disc while non-sensitive cultures will grow to the edge of the disc.

3. Paraphenylene diamine test

This test is designed to show the enzyme tyrosine decarboxylase which is involved in the synthesis of melanin pigment characteristic of *A. salmonicida*. The test is performed as soon as growth is visible (usually 24 hours) and is an indication the culture will form the brown, water-soluble pigment. The test was designed by Griffin, Snieszko and Friddle (1953) and is performed in the following manner.

a. A 1 percent aqueous solution of paraphenylene diamine (PPD) is prepared the same day it is to be used.
b. Growth on a slant or plate culture is flooded with PPD and if positive the colonies or a confluent growth will develop a brown to black color within 90 seconds.

[7]Merck and Co., Rahway, N.J. Form used in photography.

It should be emphasized that bacteria other than *A. salmonicida* will be PPD positive and this test alone is not reliable for diagnosis. However when used with other diagnostic tests the PPD is very useful in that a gram-negative non-motile PPD positive organism is usually *A. salmonicida.*

4. Motility

Motility by means of flagella may be determined by:

a. Inoculation of the bacterium into a stab of semi-soft medium such as Motility Sulfide Medium (Difco) and observing to see if growth moves out from the inoculum.

b. By direct observation of bacteria in a hanging drop. Hanging drop preparation is described in all texts on bacteriological methods. Once the slide is prepared the observer should find the edge of the drop under low power and then switch over to high dry (43X) magnification for determination of motility. Brownian-movement may often be mistaken for motility. However this may be overcome by remembering that in true motility the cells move from place to place but with Brownian movement cells vibrate in one spot and do not move.

*Serodiagnostic methods*

The use of diagnostic serological tests for identification of bacterial and other pathogens has been used extensively in human medicine and is now being used to some extent in fish pathology.

Diagnostic antisera may be obtained from commercial sources or prepared by the investigator. Rabbits are usually used for this purpose and there are many different methods of rabbit immunization and serum preparation described in textbooks. The procedure which is employed in this laboratory with satisfactory results is as follows.

Generally either a whole cell or cell-free extract antigen is used.

a. Preparation of whole cell antigens for agglutination test:
The culture is checked for purity and then grown on agar medium in Blake Bottles (usually 2 bottles per each antigen) until good growth is obtained. The growth is then washed off with 0.9% NaCl and the suspension centrifuged. The cells are washed four times in saline and resuspended in 10–20 milliliters saline or in enough saline to give a heavy cell suspension. The suspension is heated for 1 hour at 65°C to kill bacterial cells.

b. Cell-free extract antigen for agar gel precipitin test.
Culture is prepared as for whole cell antigen through the washing procedure. The wet cells are then disrupted by sonication, other mechanical ways or by manual grinding. Disruption by grinding may be achieved by transferring the wet cell pack to a mortar and then grinding for 10–15 minutes with fine carborundum. Saline (10–20 milliliters) is then added and the suspension centrifuged. The super-

natant is collected and heated for 1 hour at 65°C to detoxify the freed endotoxins.

*Rabbit immunization*

Rabbits are immunized (at least two per antigen) by initially injecting 0.5 milliliter of the antigen intravenously via the marginal ear vein. This is followed by weekly injections until the antibody titer is satisfactory (usually 6–8 weeks). In order to avoid anaphylactic shock, rabbits should be desensitized after the initial injection. This may be done by injecting 0.1 milliliter of the antigen intraperitoneally, waiting 2–4 hours and then giving the usual amount of antigen intravenously. For bleed-out rabbits are anesthetized by intraperitoneal injection of 5% pentobarbital and bled by cardiac puncture. Antiserum is separated by centrifugation and preserved by freezing.

*Slide agglutination test*

After 18–24 hours incubation, pick 1–2 colonies from the initial isolation plate culture, mix with saline and place 2 drops of the cell-saline suspension on a slide. Add 1 drop of antiserum to 1 drop and saline to the other. Agglutination of bacterial cells in antiserum but not in saline indicates a positive agglutination.

*Double diffusion precipitin test in agar gel (Ouchterlony)*

At present the agar gel precipitin test is used to identify *A. liquefaciens* and some oxidative pseudomonads. It was found that rabbit antisera prepared from a cell-free extract culture of *A. liquefaciens* and tested with gram-negative cultures representing several genera, formed precipitin bands only with members of the *Aeromonas* genus. Since *A. salmonicida* may be readily identified by slide agglutination test, the precipitin test has been useful in identifying the motile aeromonads considered here as one species, *A. liquefaciens*. The procedure is as follows:

a. Prepare agar gel diffusion plates (as suggested at the end of this section) or use commercially prepared plates. Good results have been obtained with immuno-plates pattern G[8].

b. Pipette antiserum in center well and antigens to be tested in peripheral wells. In practice, antigen for each culture is prepared by washing off the growth from a 24–48 hour slant culture with 0.3–0.5 milliliter of 0.9% saline.

c. Store the immuno plate at room temperature and examine daily. Results are usually obtained after 24 hours. The formation of one or more precipitin bands (Fig. 9) is a positive reaction.

Many cultures of *A. liquefaciens* will form several bands, some of which are continuous with each other, indicating a close serological relationship.

[8]Hyland, Division of Travenol Lab., Inc., Los Angeles, California.

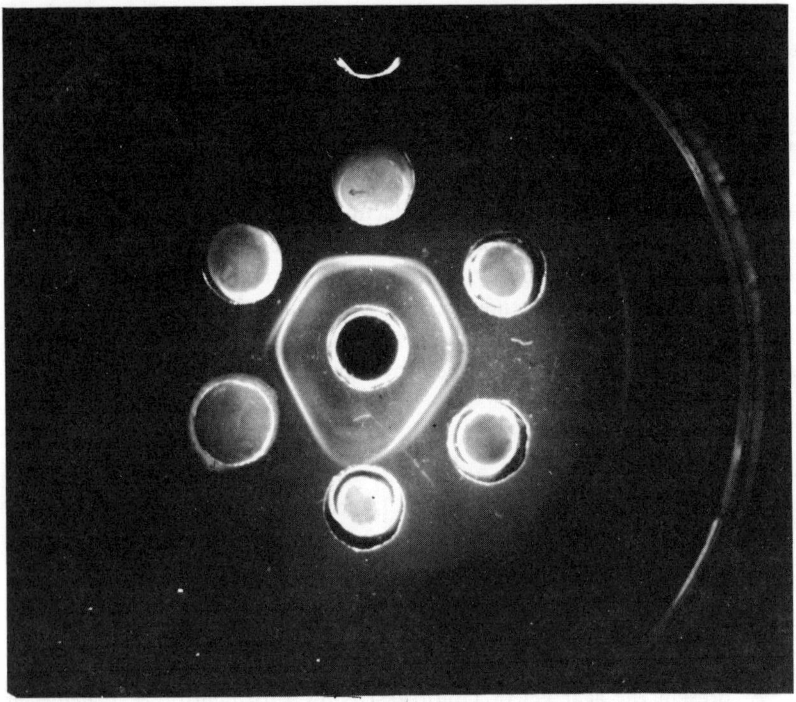

Figure 9. Demonstration of precipitin bands by agar gel diffusion. Photograph taken with plus six close-up lens. (Bullock, 1966.)

However for diagnostic purposes, one need only note formation of one or more precipitin bands.

*Non-nutritive medium for agar gel diffusion* (Bullock, 1966)

Tests may be carried out in 60 millimeter Petri plates containing 7 milliliters of the following medium:

| | |
|---|---|
| LKB[9] Veronal Barbital Buffer Stock Sol. | 25.0 ml |
| Washed Noble Agar[10] | 1.0 gm |
| Thimerosal | 0.01 gm |
| Deionized water | 75.0 ml |
| pH | 8.5 |

A phosphate buffered medium (pH 7.2) was also tested and gave comparable results, however, the barbiturate buffered medium has been used extensively. Noble agar was prepared by washing several times in deionized water, twice in 95 percent ethanol, once in acetone and then dried before use.

A pattern consisting of a 5 millimeter central well for antiserum and six surrounding wells for antigens (Fig. 10) is used for precipitin testing. The

[9]LKB-Produkter, Stockholm 12, Sweden.

[10]Difco Laboratories, Inc., Detroit, Michigan.

pattern is cut in the hardened agar by placing each plate over a template, cutting each well with a cork borer, and removing the agar plugs with a Pasteur pipette fitted with a suction hose. A drop of melted agar is placed in the bottom of each well to avoid leakage of antigen or antiserum. A well is cut on the periphery of the plate for orientation and wells number 1–6 (Fig. 10).

**Other useful chemicals for examination of fish**

ANAESTHETICS

Quinaldine (2 methylquinoline)
Eastman Kodak Co.
Distillation Products Industries
Eastman Organic Chemicals Dept.
Rochester, N.Y. 14603
1:20,000 should kill fish in a few minutes.

Figure 10. Agar gel diffusion plate showing peripheral orientation well; antigen wells 1–6, and central antiserum well. Photograph taken with plus three close-up lens. (Bullock, 1966).

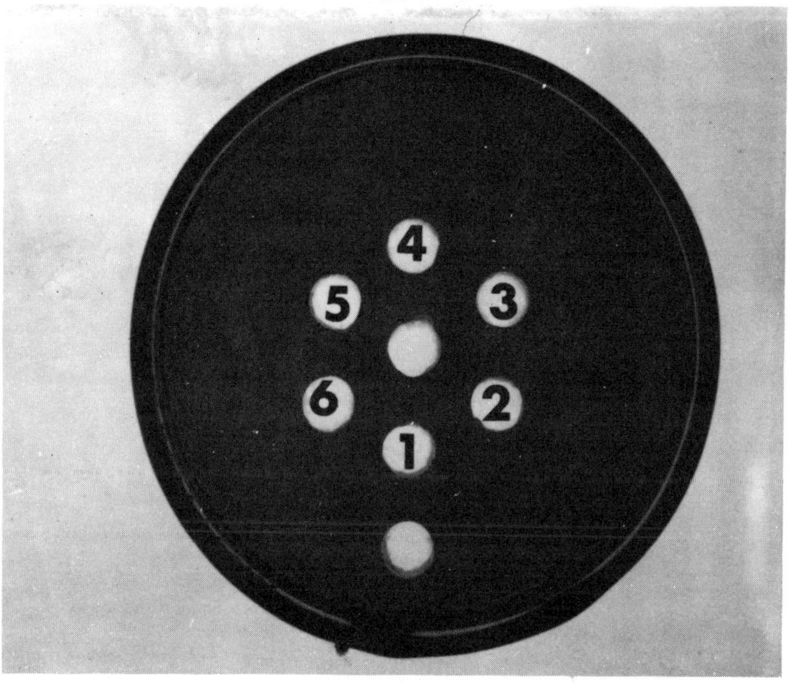

MS–222 (tricaine methanesulfonate)
Sandoz Pharmaceuticals, Ltd.
Dorval, P.Q., Canada
Hanover, N.J.
1:1000 should kill fish in a few minutes.

(Note: Availability of MS–222 is restricted by regulations.)

DISINFECTANTS

Many substances such as household bleach are suitable external disinfectants for fish. Follow directions on the label.

Quarternary ammonium compounds such as Roccal[11] (Benzalkonium chloride) used at a concentration of 1:1000 of active ingredient is very satisfactory.

[11]Sterwin Chemicals, Industrial Chemicals Division, Subsidiary of Sterling Drug, Inc., New York, N.Y.

## REFERENCES


Adams, J. N. and N. M. McClung. 1960. Morphological studies in the genus *Nocardia*. V. Septation in *Nocardia rubra* and *Jensenia canicruria*. J. Bacteriol. 80 : 281–282.

Adams, J. N. and N. M. McClung. 1962. Comparison of the developmental cycles of some members of the genus *Nocardia*. J. Bacteriol. 84 : 206–216.

Allen, N. and M. Pelczar. 1967. Bacteriological studies on the white perch *Roccus americanus*. Chesapeak Sci. 8 : 135–154.

Anacker, R. L. and E. J. Ordal. 1955. Studies on the myxobacterium *Chondrococcus columnaris*. I. Serological typing. J. Bacteriol. 78 : 25–32.

Bojalil, L. F. and J. Cerbón. 1961. Taxonomic analysis of non-pigmented, rapidly growing mycobacteria. J. Bacteriol. 81 : 338–345.

Borg. A. 1948. Studies on myxobacteria associated with diseases in salmonid fishes. Thesis. Univ. Washington, Seattle. 162 p.

Borg, A. 1960. Studies on myxobacteria associated with diseases in salmonid fishes. Wildl. Dis. 8 : 1–85. (2 microcards).

Bisset, K. 1946. The effect of temperature on non-specific infections in fish. J. Pathol. Bacteriol. 58 : 251–258.

Bisset, K. 1948. Seasonal changes in the normal flora of freshwater fish. J. Hyg. 46 : 94–97.

Breed, R. S., E. G. D. Murray and N. R. Smith. 1957. Bergey's Manual of Determinative Bacteriology. Seventh Edition, Williams and Wilkins Co., Baltimore. 1094 p.

Buck, J. D., S. P. Meyers and E. Leifson. 1963. *Pseudomonas (Flavobacterium) piscicida* Bein comb. nov. J. Bacteriol. 86 : 1125–1126.

Bullock, G. L. 1965. Characteristics and pathogenicity of a capsulated *Pseudomonas* isolated from goldfish. Appl. Microbiol. 13 : 89–92.

Bullock, G. L. 1966. Precipitin and agglutinin reactions of aeromonads isolated from fish and other sources. Bull. Off. Int. Epiz. 65 : 805–824.

Bullock, G. L. and S. F. Snieszko. 1969. Bacteria in the blood and kidney of apparently healthy hatchery trout. Amer. Fish Soc., Trans. 98 : 268–271.

Carlson, R. V. and R. E. Pacha. 1968. Procedure for the isolation and enumeration of myxobacteria from aquatic habitats. Appl. Microbiol. 16 : 795–796.

Cowan, S. T. and K. J. Steel, 1965. Manual for the Identification of Medical Bacteria . Cambridge Univ. Press, Cambridge, England. 217 p.

Davis, G. H. G. and R. W. A. Park. 1962. A taxonomic study of certain bacteria currently classified as Vibrio species. J. Gen. Microbiol. 27 : 101–119.

Evelyn, T. P. T. and L. A. McDermott. 1961. Bacteriological studies of freshwater fish. I. Isolation of aerobic bacteria from several species of Ontario fish. Can. J. Microbiol. 7 : 375–382.

Gordon, R. E. 1966. Some strains in search of a genus—*Corynebacterium, Mycobacterium, Nocardia* or what? J. Gen. Microbiol. 43 : 329–343.

Gordon, R. E. and J. M. Mihm. 1957. A comparative study of some strains received as Nocardiae. J. Bacteriol. 73 : 15–27.

Gordon, Ruth E. and Joan M. Mihm 1962. The type species of the genus *Nocardia.* J. Gen. Microbiol. 27 : 1–10.
Griffin, P. J., S. F. Snieszko and S. B. Friddle. 1953. A new adjuvant in the diagnosis of fish furunculosis caused by *Bacterium salmonicida.* Vet. Med. 48 : 280–282.
Hoshina, T. 1957. Further observations on the causative bacteria of the epidemic disease-like furunculosis of rainbow trout. J. Tokyo Univ. Fish. 43 : 59–66.
Janssen, W. A. and M. T. Surgalla. 1968. Morphology, physiology and, serology of a *Pasteurella* species, pathogenic for white perch *(Roccus americanus)*. J. Bacteriol. 96 : 1606–1610.
Jones, R. J. and D. E. Jenkins. 1965. Mycobacteria isolated from soil. Can. J. Microbiol. 11 : 127–133.
Klontz, G. W. and D. P. Anderson. 1968. Fluorescent antibody studies of isolates of *Aeromonas salmonicida.* Bull. Off. Int. Epiz. 69 : 1149–1157.
Leifson, E. 1961. The effect of formaldehyde on the shape of bacterial flagella. J. Gen. Microbiol. 25 : 131–133.
Manion, R., S. Bradley, H. Zinneman and W. Hall. 1964. Interrelationships among mycobacteria and Nocardiae. J. Bacteriol. 87 : 1056–1059.
Novel, E. 1939. Une technique facile et rapide de mise en evidence des cils bacteriens. Ann. Inst. Pasteur 63 : 302–311.
Ordal, E. J. and B. J. Earp. 1956. Cultivation and transmission of etiological agent of kidney disease in salmonid fishes. Soc. Exp. Biol. Med., Proc. 92 : 85–88.
Pacha, R. E. 1968. Characteristics of *Cytophaga psychrophila* (Borg) isolated during outbreaks of bacterial cold-water disease. Appl. Microbiol. 16 : 97–101.
Parisot, Thomas, J. 1958. Tuberculosis of fish. A review of the literature with a description of the disease in salmonid fish. Bacteriol. Rev. 22 : 240–245.
Rabb, L., J. W. Cornick and L. A. McDermott. 1964. A macroscopic-slide agglutination test for the presumptive diagnosis of furunculosis in fish. Prog. Fish-Cult. 26 : 118–120.
Robinson, J. and F. Meyer. 1966. Streptococcal fish pathogen. J. Bacteriol. 92 : 512.
Ross, A. J., R. R. Rucker and W. H. Ewing. 1966. Description of a bacterium associated with redmouth disease of rainbow trout (*Salmo gairdneri*). Can. J. Microbiol. 12 : 763–770.
Saito, Y., M. Otsuru, T. Furukawa, K. Kanda and A. Sato. 1964. Studies on an infectious disease of rainbow trout. Acta Med. Biol. 11 : 267–295.
Sakazaki, R., S. Iwanami, and H. Fukumi. 1963. Studies on the enteropathogenic, facultative halophilic bacteria *Vibrio parahaemolyticus.* I. Morphological, cultural and biochemical properties and its taxonomical position. Jap. J. Med. Sci. Biol. 16 : 161–188.
Schubert, R. H. W. 1962. Zur Technik der Differenzierung von Vibrionen und Pseudomonaden mit dem Vibriostaticum 0/129. Zentralbl. Bakteriol. Parasitenk. Infekt. Hyg. 184 : 560–561.
Sherris, J. C. 1963. Some recent advances in diagnostic medical bacteriology. Ann. Rev. Microbiol. 17 : 565–592.

Shewan, J. M. 1963. The differentiation of certain genera of gram-negative bacteria frequently encountered in marine environments. *In* Symposium on Marine Microbiology. Compiled and edited by Carl H. Oppenheimer. Charles C. Thomas publisher, Springfield, Ill. 499–521.

Simidu, U. and K. Hasuo. 1968a. An improved medium for the isolation of bacteria from marine fish. J. Gen. Microbiol. 52 : 355–360.

Simidu, U. and K. Hasuo. 1968b. Salt dependency of the bacterial flora of marine fish. J. Gen. Microbiol. 52 : 347–354.

Skerman, V. B. D. 1967. A Guide to the Identification of the Genera of Bacteria. Second Edition, Williams and Wilkins Co., Baltimore. 303 p.

Smith, I. W. 1964. The occurrence and pathology of Dee disease. Freshwater and Salmon Fish. Res. 34 : 1–12.

Snieszko, S. F., G. L. Bullock, E. Hollis and J. G. Boone. 1964. *Pasteurella* sp. from an epizootic of white perch *(Roccus americanus)* in Chesapeake Bay Tidewater Areas. J. Bacteriol. 88 : 1814–1815

Society of American Bacteriologists. 1957. Manual of Microbiological Methods. McGraw-Hill Co., New York. 315 p.

Zamora, A., L. F. Bojalil and F. Bastarrachea. 1963. Immunologically active polysaccharides from *Nocardia asteroides* and *Nocardia brasiliensis*. J. Bacteriol. 85 : 549–555.

# INDEX

*IDENTIFICATION OF FISH PATHOGENIC BACTERIA,*
*Supplemental Color Plates.*

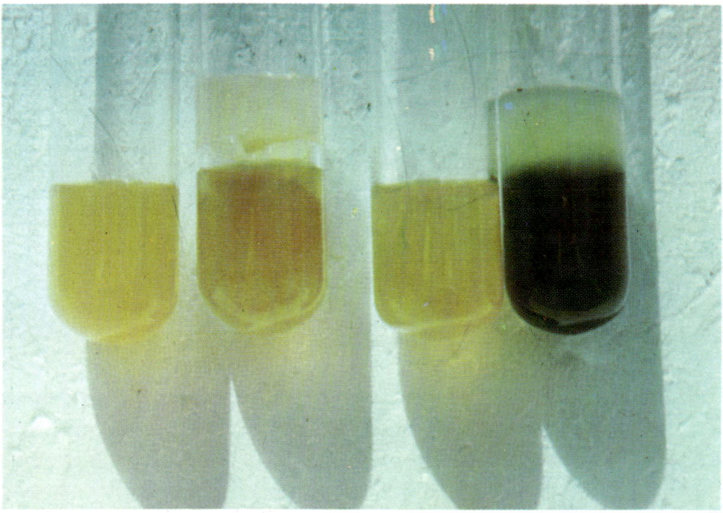

Figure 7. Oxidation and fermentation reactions in o/f glucose. The two tubes on the right show oxidation; the two tubes on the left show aerogenic fermentation.
See page *31*

Figure 8. Cytochrome oxidase test using impregnated paper strip. Positive test indicated by blue color.

See page *33*